1984

D1084488

# PHARYNGITIS

# PHARYNGITIS
Management in an Era
of Declining Rheumatic Fever

Edited by

## Stanford T. Shulman, M.D.

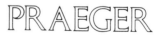

PRAEGER SPECIAL STUDIES • PRAEGER SCIENTIFIC

New York • Philadelphia • Eastbourne, UK
Toronto • Hong Kong • Tokyo • Sydney

Library of Congress Cataloging in Publication Data

Main entry under title:

Pharyngitis: management in an era of declining rheumatic
    fever.

    "Based in part on a conference held 16-19 February
1983, sponsored by Ross Laboratories"—T.p. verso.
    Includes index.
    1. Pharyngitis—Congresses.    2. Rheumatic fever—Com-
plications and sequelae—Congresses.    I. Shulman,
Stanford T.    II. Ross Laboratories. (DNLM: 1. Pharyngitis
—Therapy—Congresses.    2. Pharyngitis—Complications—
Congresses.    3. Streptococcal infections—Complications—
Congresses.    4. Rheumatic fever—Etiology—Congresses.
WV 410 P536    1983)
RF485.P43    1984        616.3'2        83-26897
ISBN 0-03-062957-8 (alk. paper)

*To Claire, Debbie, Liz, Ed, Esther and
Sam, and my mother for their support
and love, and to the Infectious Disease
group for their assistance and counsel.*

Published in 1984 by Praeger Publishers
CBS Educational and Professional Publishing
a Division of CBS Inc.

© 1984 by Praeger Publishers

456789    052    987654321

Printed in the United States of America
on acid-free paper.

# Dedication

This volume is dedicated to Dr. Lewis W. Wannamaker (1923-1983), whose untimely death occurred on 25 March 1983, shortly after his participation in the proceedings that led to this work.

Dr. Wannamaker was born in St. Mathews, North Carolina. He was graduated from Emory University with a B.A. in 1943 and from Duke University's School of Medicine with his M.D. in 1946. He took his training in general pediatrics at Duke and in 1947 started a fellowship in Infectious Diseases. It was shortly thereafter that Lewis Wannamaker was introduced to the world of streptococcus, a world he lived in for the remainder of his life. For in 1948, he joined a special group of individuals at Warren Air Force Base, Wyoming, that included Floyd Denny, William Brink, Hal Houser, and later Al Stetson and others, all of whom were recruited to work with the dynamic and inspiring Charles Rammelkamp.

The work generated by this group produced some of the most fundamental knowledge regarding the relationship of the group A streptococcus to rheumatic fever and to nephritis, the epidemiology of these diseases, and above all, the effect of treatment of streptococcal pharyngitis on the prevention of rheumatic fever. It was in the latter area that Lewis W. Wannamaker, as first author of a manuscript entitled "Prophylaxis of Acute Rheumatic Fever," published in the *American Journal of Medicine* in June 1951, made one of his initial and most compelling contributions.

In subsequent years, Dr. Wannamaker continued a most productive career. His work on the streptococcal DNAses with Dr. Maclyn McCarty and his observations on the relationship of throat and skin infection to rheumatic fever and nephritis were some of the important contributions that resulted in over two hundred independent publications. These original contributions deserved many recognitions and awards, which included a Lifetime Career Investigatorship of the American Heart Association, the Alexander von Humboldt Foundation Senior Scientist Award, The Robert Koch Prize and Medal, and election to membership of the National Academy of Science.

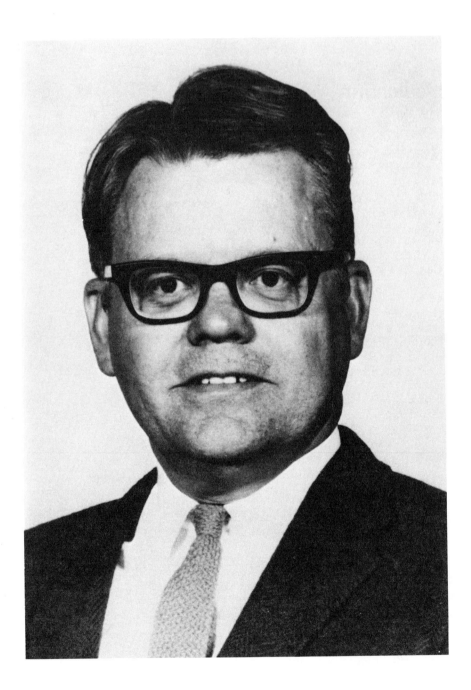

More important yet is the legacy of those scientists who had the unique opportunity of working with him for several years. All of us, Paul Quie, Hugh Dillon, Bud Anthony, Carolyn Hardegree, Don Amren, Ken Dunnor, Waleed Yasmineh, Steven Skjold, John Matson, Franklin Top, Jr., Ron Shapira, Joe Brown, John Tagg, Leslie Benchetrit, John Hill, Warren Regelmann, Ernie Gray, Adnan Dajani, Patricia Ferrieri, Ed Kaplan, Burt Dudding, Harry Hill, Joe Ferretti, Mike Gerber, David Speert, and myself, who were privileged to work directly with him, and the many others who were directly or indirectly touched by his life, are saddened by his untimely departure. We, along with his family and his friends, will miss him. We will miss his advice, his wisdom, his dogged and meticulous honesty in his work, his tolerance, his congeniality, and above all, his love to us and to his fellow man.

—*Elia M. Ayoub, M.D.*
Professor of Pediatrics
University of Florida
Gainesville, Florida

# Contents

# List of Contributors

*Don P. Amren, M.D.*
Pediatrician,
St. Louis Park Medical Center,
Clinical Professor of Pediatrics,
University of Minnesota Hospitals, Minneapolis.

*Bascom F. Anthony, M.D.*
Professor of Pediatrics,
Chief, Pediatric Infectious Diseases,
Harbor-UCLA Medical Center,
University of California at Los Angeles,
School of Medicine, Torrance.

*Elia M. Ayoub, M.D.*
Professor of Pediatrics,
Chief, Division of Infectious
Disease and Immunology,
University of Florida, Gainesville.

*Robert S. Baltimore, M.D.*
Associate Professor,
Departments of Pediatrics and
Epidemiology,
Yale University School of Medicine,
New Haven, Connecticut.

*Marc O. Beem, M.D.*
Professor of Pediatrics,
Chief, Pediatric Infectious Diseases,
Pritzker School of Medicine,
University of Chicago, Illinois.

*Alan L. Bisno, M.D.*
Professor of Internal Medicine,
Chief, Division of Infectious Diseases,
Department of Medicine,
University of Tennessee Center
for the Health Sciences, Memphis.

*Stephen L. Cochi, M.D.*
EIS Officer, Epidemiology Section,
Respiratory and Special
Pathogens Branch,
Division of Bacterial Diseases,
Center for Infectious Diseases,
Centers for Disease Control,
Atlanta, Georgia.

*Adnan S. Dajani, M.D.*

Professor of Pediatrics,
Wayne State University,
Director, Division of Infectious Diseases,
Children's Hospital of Michigan, Detroit.

*Charles P. Darby, M.D.*

Professor and Chairman,
Department of Pediatrics,
Medical University of South Carolina,
Charleston.

*Jeffrey P. Davis, M.D.*

State Epidemiologist,
Chief, Section of Acute and
Communicable Disease Epidemiology,
Wisconsin Division of Health,
Adjunct Assistant Professor,
Departments of Preventive Medicine
and Pediatrics,
University of Wisconsin School
of Medicine, Madison.

*Floyd W. Denny, M.D.*

Professor of Pediatrics,
University of North Carolina,
Chapel Hill.

*Hugh C. Dillon, Jr., M.D.*

Professor of Pediatrics and
Microbiology,
University of Alabama School
of Medicine, Birmingham.

*David T. Durack, D.Phil., M.D.*

Professor of Medicine,
Chief, Infectious Diseases,
Department of Medicine,
Duke University Medical Center,
Durham, North Carolina.

*Robert Edelman, M.D.*

Chief, Clinical and Epidemiological
Studies Branch,
National Institute of Allergy
and Infectious Diseases,
National Institutes of Health,
Bethesda, Maryland.

*Theodore C. Eickhoff, M.D.*

Director of Internal Medicine,
Presbyterian/St. Luke's
Medical Center,
Professor of Medicine,
University of Colorado
School of Medicine, Denver.

Richard R. Facklam, Ph.D.    Chief, Reference Bacteriology
Section,
Respiratory and Special
Pathogens Branch,
Division of Bacterial Diseases,
Center for Infectious Diseases,
Centers for Disease Control,
Atlanta, Georgia.

Alvan R. Feinstein, M.D.    Professor of Medicine and
Epidemiology,
Director, Clinical Epidemiology Unit,
Yale University School of Medicine,
New Haven, Connecticut.

Patricia Ferrieri, M.D.    Professor of Pediatrics and
Laboratory Medicine/Pathology,
University of Minnesota Medical School,
Minneapolis.

Ben R. Forsyth, M.D.    Professor of Medicine and Medical
Microbiology,
University of Vermont
College of Medicine,
Burlington.

Michael A. Gerber, M.D.    Assistant Professor of Pediatrics,
University of Connecticut
Health Center,
Farmington.

Leon Gordis, M.D., Dr.P.H.    Professor and Chairman,
Department of Epidemiology,
The Johns Hopkins University
School of Hygiene and Public Health,
Baltimore, Maryland.

Harry R. Hill, M.D.    Professor of Pathology and
Pediatrics,
University of Utah School
of Medicine,
Salt Lake City.

Harold B. Houser, M.D.    Professor of Epidemiology,
Chairman, Department of Biometry,
School of Medicine,
Case Western Reserve University,
Cleveland, Ohio.

*William S. Jordan, Jr., M.D.*    Director, Microbiology and
Infectious Diseases Program,
National Institute of Allergy
and Infectious Diseases,
National Institutes of Health,
Bethesda, Maryland.

*Edward L. Kaplan, M.D.*    Professor of Pediatrics,
University of Minnesota
School of Medicine, Minneapolis.

*Anthony L. Komaroff, M.D.*  Associate Professor of Medicine,
Harvard Medical School,
Boston, Massachusetts.

*Mack Land, M.D.*    Division of Infectious Diseases,
The University of Tennessee,
Center for the Health Sciences,
Memphis, Tennessee.

*Milton Markowitz, M.D.*    Professor and Head,
Department of Pediatrics,
University of Connecticut Health Center,
Farmington.

*Maclyn McCarty, M.D.*    Professor Emeritus,
Rockefeller University,
New York, New York.

*H. Dean Millard, D.D.S., M.S.*    Professor and Chairman,
Department of Oral Diagnosis
and Radiology,
The University of Michigan
School of Dentistry,
Ann Arbor.

*Edward A. Mortimer, Jr., M.D.*    Professor and Chairman,
Department of Epidemiology
and Community Health,
Professor of Pediatrics,
School of Medicine,
Case Western Reserve University,
Cleveland, Ohio.

*Robert H. Pantell, M.D.*    Associate Professor and Director,
Division of General Pediatrics,
University of California,
San Francisco.

*Jay P. Sanford, M.D.*                    President and Dean,
School of Medicine, Professor of Medicine,
Uniformed Services University
of the Health Sciences, Bethesda, Maryland.

*Richard H. Schwartz, M.D.*    Clinical Associate Professor for
Child Health and Development,
Clinical Associate Professor of Pediatrics,
Georgetown University School of Medicine,
Washington, D.C.

*Stanford T. Shulman, M.D.*          Professor of Pediatrics,
Northwestern University Medical School,
Chief, Pediatric Infectious Diseases,
The Children's Memorial Hospital,
Chicago.

*Gene H. Stollerman, M.D.*           Professor of Medicine,
Department of Internal Medicine,
Boston University School of Medicine,
Massachusetts.

*Angelo Taranta, M.D.*                Director of Medicine
Cabrini Medical Center,
New York, New York,
Professor of Medicine, Chief,
Rheumatology/Immunology Section,
New York Medical College, Valhalla.

*Richard K. Tompkins, M.D.*       Professor of Medicine and
Health Sciences,
University of Washington,
Executive Director,
Seattle Public Health Hospital,
Washington.

*Lewis W. Wannamaker, M.D.*       Professor of Pediatrics and
Microbiology,
University of Minnesota Medical School,
Minneapolis.

*John A. Washington II, M.D.*       Head, Section of Clinical
Microbiology,
Mayo Clinic,
Professor of Microbiology
and Laboratory Medicine,
Mayo Medical School,
Rochester, Minnesota.

*Chatrchai Watanakunakorn, M.D.*            Professor of Internal
Medicine,
Chief, Infectious Diseases,
Northeastern Ohio Universities,
College of Medicine, Youngstown.

# Preface

*Stanford T. Shulman, M.D.*

The apparent dramatic change in the incidence of acute rheumatic fever in the United States in recent years, and the possible implications of this change for strategies of management of the patient with pharyngitis, stimulated the American Heart Association's Committee on Rheumatic Fever and Bacterial Endocarditis to organize a conference on the topic, "Management of Pharyngitis in an Era of Declining Rheumatic Fever." With support and funding graciously provided by Ross Laboratories and its Director of Professional Services, Mr. Dewey Sehring, plus the endorsement of the National Institute of Allergy and Infectious Diseases, an organizing committee—composed of Drs. Milton Markowitz, Edward Kaplan, Alan Bisno, Floyd Denny, Leon Gordis, and me—invited a panel of leading clinical investigators to assemble for two days of presentations and discussions focused on various aspects of the epidemiology, diagnosis, and management of pharyngitis.

Although the presentations and vigorous related discussions that occurred over these two days in February 1983 will form the basis for the next revision of the American Heart Association's statement, "Prevention of Rheumatic Fever," and although an abridged version of the conference proceedings has been published by Ross Laboratories, the present volume is offered as an unabridged permanent record of the meeting. The importance of the topic—one of the most common reasons that patients seek medical care (third only to well care and obstetrical visits)—and the high quality of the presentations and discussions presented here in their entirety would, by themselves, fully justify publication of this book. However, this volume in addition includes four invited papers, prepared after the conference and commissioned specifically for this book, by Drs. Edward Mortimer and Harold Houser, John Washington, Angelo Taranta, and Floyd Denny. These contributions, from distinguished representatives of the disciplines of Epidemiology, Clinical Microbiology, Medicine and Rheumatology, and Pediatrics and Infectious Diseases, respectively, provide unique after-the-fact reflections that place the proceedings in a larger context.

As noted above, this book addresses the truly remarkable, inexplicable decline, over the past one to two decades, in the incidence in the United States of acute rheumatic fever, a disease once considered a major medical disorder in this country. Even as we hasten to acknowledge that rheumatic fever and rheumatic heart disease persist as serious problems in many less developed areas of the world and that the data and opinions expressed in this book are not applicable to these other regions, we nevertheless must view the dramatic decline of acute rheumatic fever in the U.S. as another milestone in the history of the group A streptococcus. This preface would not be complete, then, without a brief recapitulation of some of the other milestones in the history of this organism: In the late 15th Century, St. Anthony's Chapel was erected in Edinburgh, Scotland, for sufferers of "St. Anthony's fire" (erysipelas), a major cause of mortality at that time. The ruins of this chapel still stand. In 1874, the Viennese surgeon Theodor Billroth first applied the term "streptococcus" to the chain-forming cocci that he observed microscopically in cases of erysipelas and infected wounds. Five years later, Louis Pasteur described cocci in chains in the blood of a patient with puerperal sepsis; and shortly thereafter, he produced streptococcal septicemia in rabbits inoculated with human saliva. In 1884, ninety-nine years ago, the current name, *Streptococcus pyogenes*, was introduced by Rosenbach for the chain-forming cocci that he isolated from suppurative lesions of man. The remarkable studies of the late Dr. Rebecca Lancefield, which spanned more than a half-century, established the basis for the serologic grouping of streptococci. Certainly Sir Alexander Fleming's discovery of penicillin in 1929, leading to the use of penicillin in man, beginning in 1941 at the Radcliffe Infirmary in Oxford, also was an important milestone in the history of the streptococcus.

Finally, today—forty-two years after the introduction of penicillin—the contributors to this monograph examine the implications of the virtual disappearance of acute rheumatic fever from medical practice in the United States. While it would be presumptuous to consider publication of this book as still another milestone, I hope that epidemiologists, microbiologists, and clinicians will find the data and discussions presented here to be stimulating and informative.

—*Stanford T. Shulman, M.D.*

# Part One:
# The Conference Proceedings

# Preview of Controversial Issues

*Milton Markowitz, M.D.*

I would like to begin by sharing with you a letter I recently received from a physician in Connecticut:

Dear Doctor Markowitz,

For the past decade or more, a great deal has been written in the medical literature and the lay press about the prevention of rheumatic fever. Your interest in this disease and your connection with American Heart Association programs prompt me to write to raise some questions regarding the recommendations which you are promoting in Connecticut.

To help me support my thesis, I have reviewed my experience with rheumatic fever during the past 15 years. During this period I have seen six proven cases. Could I have prevented these attacks? In the first place, three of these six children were not seen by me prior to their rheumatic episode either because they had no sore throat symptoms or they did not choose to seek my advice. Therefore, there were only three cases, or about one case every five years, which in theory could have been prevented. I say theoretically because there are respected people in New England who do not believe that first attacks of rheumatic fever can be prevented. I know you consider this to be heresy, so let us assume the data obtained in young adults are applicable to children.

Now let us look at what might have been required to prevent this one case of rheumatic fever during the five-year period. Although I do not have precise figures, I must see at least 1,000 children a year with complaints and/or physical findings indicative of pharyngitis. This would mean 5,000 throat cultures over a five-year period. It is likely that 30% of these patients with pharyngitis would have had a positive culture and therefore would be required to return for another culture after treatment. This adds another 1,500 cultures. Furthermore, were I to follow the current recommendations and culture family contacts, 3,000 additional throat swabs would be required—for a grand total of approximately 10,000 cultures over this five-year period. Consider, if you will, the cost of this streptococcal witch hunt in energy, time, and money. Currently the State Health Department processes 250,000 cultures per year at a cost of $250,000. Would not this cost be increased at least ten-fold if only the majority of, let alone all, physicians used throat culture extensively?

Mind you, I appreciate the value of throat culture in some patients and I have been using this procedure more frequently than I did in the past. However, I am concerned when I see young physicians being trained to culture virtually every respiratory infection, almost without regard for the history and physical findings. I deplore this trend to over-utilize laboratory procedures, and I believe many patients are being treated needlessly on the basis of culture findings only. I also believe we are producing unnecessary anxiety in families, especially in those patients who carry streptococci for weeks and even months. Not infrequently, this anxiety provokes parents to seek a tonsillectomy, which might otherwise have been avoided.

Regarding streptococcal carriage, is it not true that persistence of these organisms in the pharynx stimulates more solid immunity? If so, and if as I believe, rheumatic fever is not a significant problem in my practice, might not my patients be better served by a short course of treatment, or perhaps no treatment at all, if the illness is very mild? In truth, most patients probably only receive a three to five-day course of treatment, and yet we still see so little rheumatic fever. I am reminded that I began practice in 1937, and while I do not have exact figures, I do not recall having a significant number of private patients with rheumatic fever in the ten years before penicillin became available. Is it not possible that we need different recommendations for children who are at very low risk for rheumatic fever? After all, I do not screen for lead poisoning in my patients who live in the suburbs, yet it is certainly a valid procedure for children who live in the inner city.

Finally, I should tell you that among my six rheumatic fever cases, there is only one with residual heart disease. The disease is milder and we can protect against recurrent attacks. Therefore, it may be less important to prevent first attacks, considering the cumbersome and imperfect means available to us at this time.

I would appreciate your thoughts on the questions I have raised.

Sincerely yours,
*Marcus Welby, M.D.*


THIRTY YEARS WAR AGAINST THE STREPTOCOCCUS:
AN HISTORICAL PERSPECTIVE

Physicians who received their clinical training or practiced pediatrics prior to 1950 rarely bothered to determine the etiology of pharyngitis unless diphtheria was suspected. In general, throat cultures were reserved for hospitalized patients. While streptococcal pharyngitis has been recognized as a specific clinical entity for more than sixty years [1], until relatively recently, it did not receive any special attention unless it was accompanied by a scarlatiniform rash. In fact, prior to 1951, the American Academy of Pediatrics' Bible on infectious diseases, the "Red Book," made no mention of this disease [2]. The availability of penicillin following World War II even enhanced this apparent complacency regarding streptococcal pharyngitis. Virtually every patient with an upper respiratory tract infection was treated with an antimicrobial agent for three to five days on the assumption that they either had a bacterial infection or that a bacterial complication could be prevented. This was the state of the art in 1950. That year marked the beginning of what I have chosen to call "the thirty years war against the streptococcus."

What I propose to do in this introduction is review briefly the changes in our approach to the management of streptococcal pharyngitis over the past three decades. The first of these decades was marked by discoveries of new information. The diagnostic and therapeutic strategies derived from this knowledge were implemented during the next decade and for the most part are adhered to. However, over the past ten years, some of these strategies have come under increasing scrutiny. A number of controversial issues have emerged that require examination.

## Decade of Discovery: 1950–60

The single most important discovery in the initiation of the war against the streptococcus was the finding by Dr. Charles Rammelkamp and his colleagues that the *initial* attack of rheumatic fever could be prevented by adequate penicillin treatment of the preceding streptococcal pharyngitis. The results of large, carefully controlled studies published by Floyd Denny et al. in 1950 [3] and by Lewis Wannamaker et al. in 1951 [4] provided the scientific basis for the recommendations that are followed to this day. This discovery was heralded as a major advance: for the first time, rheumatic heart disease—the most frequent cause of acquired heart disease in young people—could be prevented. There was now a very good reason for making a correct etiologic diagnosis and prescribing appropriate therapy for sore throats. Rheumatic heart disease became one of the very few preventable chronic diseases.

During the 1950s, practicing physicians who accepted the diagnostic challenge of identifying group A streptococcal pharyngitis soon discovered that the clinical manifestations of streptococcal pharyngitis were too variable for diagnostic accuracy. Several studies showed that even physicians with a special interest in streptococcal infections could predict the etiology of pharyngitis on clinical grounds only about half the time [5,6,7]. As methods for identifying viruses became available, it became apparent that viral infections could mimic many of the signs and symptoms of streptococcal disease, including exudate, once thought to be the single most reliable sign of streptococcal pharyngitis. Furthermore, viruses were found to be responsible for a majority of the cases of pharyngitis, while group A streptococci are responsible for 15% to 20% of endemic sore throats.

Errors in clinical diagnosis led to the use of throat cultures for bacteriologic confirmation. Dr. Burtis Breese was the first to employ this simple diagnostic tool in everyday pediatric practice [8]. He championed do-it-yourself office bacteriology to expedite results and control costs. In

1952, prompted by one of Dr. Breese's patients who had moved to Baltimore, I began doing cultures in my own practice and found them to be a valuable aid to guide clinical management.

## Decade of Dissemination: 1960–70

There is usually a considerable lag in the general implementation of any scientific advance, and it took approximately ten years before the recommendations arising from Dr. Rammelkamp's studies began to have a national impact on how sore throats were managed. The American Heart Association's campaign for the primary prevention of rheumatic fever increased the awareness among both the laity and health professionals of the importance of making an etiologic diagnosis and treating streptococcal pharyngitis appropriately. This awareness was enhanced by the fact that throughout the 1950s, physicians continued to see cases of acute rheumatic fever during their residency training. For example, at the Johns Hopkins Children's Hospital, 258 patients with acute rheumatic fever were admitted over a ten-year period, 1952–61. The hope of eradicating rheumatic fever following the introduction of preventive methods a decade earlier had clearly not been fulfilled [9].

During the 1960s, the throat culture began to be widely used to confirm clinical impressions. In many areas of the country, public health laboratories began to provide throat culture services at little or no charge to the patient. Also, many physicians followed Dr. Breese's lead and started to do bacteriology in their offices. Relatively inexpensive kits with selective media that could be used by nontechnical personnel were marketed [10].

The use of the throat culture provided considerable satisfaction for both the doctor and the patient. The physician felt that he was practicing more scientific medicine, that he could prescribe antibiotics more judiciously, and that the likelihood of compliance would be greater when the diagnosis was confirmed by a culture. The throat culture was also a legitimate source of additional income. In our practice, parents soon became accustomed to waiting for the results of throat culture before treatment was started. In about four out of five patients, the throat culture was negative and symptomatic treatment was all that was required. Parents were pleased that unnecessary antibiotic therapy had been avoided and that the cost of a culture was more than offset by saving the price of a prescription.

Thus by 1970, many practitioners were culturing virtually every patient with an upper respiratory infection and treating only those whose cultures were positive for group A beta-hemolytic streptococci. It also became fairly common practice to obtain a repeat throat culture a few days after completion of the treatment. This seemed appropriate, since it had been shown that there was a risk of rheumatic fever in patients who still had a positive culture three weeks after onset of pharyngitis [11]. Frequently, efforts were also made to detect infections among family contacts. Indeed, the 1966 edition of the "Red Book" recommended culturing household contacts of patients with streptococcal pharyngitis [12]. Searching for asymptomatic infections could be justified, since intrafamilial spread of streptococci is common and since at least one-third of patients with acute rheumatic fever give no history of a preceding pharyngitis [13].

Decade of Dissonance: 1970–80

The more liberal the indications for culturing, the greater the likelihood of detecting carriers, those individuals in whom streptococci can be found on culture but who have no other evidence of an acute streptococcal infection. Carrier rates vary with the season of the year, the socioeconomic status, the sensitivity of the bacteriologic methods, and the frequency and number of cultures taken. Unfortunately, there is no reliable way of distinguishing the carrier from the infected patient based on the culture findings. Patients with bona fide infections usually harbor large numbers of streptococci and carriers generally do not, but colony counts are not sufficiently reliable to distinguish the two conditions [14]. Since as many as 50% of patients with pharyngitis and positive cultures may be carriers [15] and since it is generally believed that carriers need no treatment, the usefulness of the throat culture as a guide to management began to be questioned.

The use of routine follow-up cultures after completion of treatment identified still another problem, that is, the failure to eradicate streptococci following a ten-day course of penicillin therapy. The rates of these bacteriologic failures are surprisingly high, ranging from 20% to 40% [16,17]. It is well established that the carrier state is difficult to eradicate, and the question here is whether these are really therapeutic failures or are patients who were carriers to begin with. It is likely that true therapeutic failures may not be all that common. However, the physician has no way of making this distinction when he is faced with a positive follow-up culture. If to prevent rheumatic fever one has to eradicate the organisms, then bona fide therapeutic failures should be re-treated. Many physicians opt for this course of action and when they do, they often find it difficult to rid the pharynx of streptococci. Not infrequently, this has led to treating asymptomatic children with numerous courses of antibiotics, often with drugs other than penicillin. This failure to eliminate streptococci after repeated treatments has also led to considerable anxiety among some parents and has created a new syndrome, "streptococcal neurosis." Many of us are consulted frequently about what Dr. Kaplan has called the "enigma of the carrier" [18]. The uncertainties created by the streptococcal carrier problem have done more to confuse the practitioner and to undermine our time-honored approach than any other issue.

Excessive culturing and unnecessary treatment of carriers have undoubtedly added considerably to the costs of managing children with pharyngitis. Indeed, the cost-effectiveness of all current efforts to prevent rheumatic fever has been the subject of much discussion and controversy. Studies using decision analysis techniques to compare the costs and outcomes of different therapeutic approaches in managing patients with pharyngitis have been published [19,20]. These will be discussed in detail later in this conference. For now, it is sufficient to note that the conclusions reached in some of these studies differ from present-day recommendations, and while they need to be carefully considered, some of the assumptions on which the conclusions have been based are difficult to verify.

Of course, the fundamental reason that the cost-effectiveness issue has been raised is that rheumatic fever has become a very uncommon disease in this country. Many physicians now go through three years of residency training without ever seeing a patient with acute rheumatic fever. Perhaps we have now reached the point where the costs and risks of preventing acute rheumatic fever are greater than the risk of acquiring the disease. However, we must first decide how much our current approach to the management of streptococcal pharyngitis actually contributed to the declining incidence of acute rheumatic fever in the United States over the past 30 years and how significant other factors have been.

SUMMARY

I shall end this brief review by posing some of the questions that I wish you would consider during the course of this meeting:

1. Should not the throat culture be used more selectively?
2. What can we do to better distinguish streptococcal carriage from infection?
3. How should asymptomatic treatment failures be managed?
4. Why are we not seeing more acute rheumatic fever?

REFERENCES

1. Felty, A. R., and A. B. Hodges. 1923. A clinical study of acute streptococcal infection of the pharyngeal lymphoid tissue. *Bull Johns Hopkins Hosp* 34:330.
2. Report of the Committee on Infectious Diseases. 1951. American Academy of Pediatrics, Evanston, Illinois.
3. Denny, F. W., L. W. Wannamaker, W. R. Brink et al. 1950. Prevention of rheumatic fever; treatment of the preceding streptococcic infection. *JAMA* 143:151.
4. Wannamaker, L. W., C. H. Rammelkamp, F. W. Denny et al. 1951. Prophylaxis of acute rheumatic fever by treatment of the preceding streptococcal infection with various amounts of depot penicillin. *Am J Med* 10:63.
5. Breese, B. B., and F. A. Disney. 1954. The accuracy of diagnosis of beta streptococcal infection on clinical grounds. *J Pediat* 44:670.
6. Siegel, A. C. 1956. The recognition of streptococcal infections in the prevention of rheumatic fever and acute glomerulonephritis. *Illinois Med J* 110:113.
7. Stillerman, M., and S. H. Bernstein. 1961. Streptococcal pharyngitis: evaluation of clinical syndromes in diagnosis. *Am J Dis Child.* 101:476.
8. Breese, B. B. 1969. Culturing beta hemolytic streptococci in pediatric practice—observations after twenty years. *J Pediat* 75:164.
9. Markowitz, M. 1970. The eradication of rheumatic fever: an unfulfilled hope. *Circulation* 41:1077.
10. Randolph, M. F., J. J. Redys, and J. Cope et al. 1976. Streptococcal pharyngitis: evaluation of a new diagnostic kit for clinic and office use. *Am J Dis Child* 130:171.
11. Cantanzaro, F. J., C. H. Rammelkamp, and R. Chamovitz. 1958. Prevention of rheumatic fever by treatment of the streptococcal infection. II. Factors responsible for failure. *New Engl J Med* 259:51.
12. Report of the Committee on Infectious Diseases, 1966. American Academy of Pediatrics, Evanston, Illinois.

13. Gordis, L., A. Lilienfeld, and R. Rodriguez. 1969. Studies on the epidemiology and preventability of rheumatic fever. *Pub Hlth Rep* 84:333.

14. Kaplan, E. L., F. H. Top, B. A. Dudding et al. 1971. Diagnosis of streptococcal pharyngitis: The problem of differentiating active infection from the carrier state in the symptomatic child. *J Infect Dis* 123:490.

15. Wannamaker, L. W. 1972. Perplexity and precision in the diagnosis of streptococcal pharyngitis. *Am J Dis Child* 124:352

16. Gastanaduy, A. S., E. L. Kaplan, B. Huwe et al. 1980. Failure of penicillin to eradicate group A. streptococci during an outbreak of pharyngitis. *Lancet* 2:498.

17. Schwartz, R. H., R. L. Wientzen, F. Pedreira et al. 1981. Penicillin V for group A streptococcal pharyngotonsillitis. *JAMA* 246:1790.

18. Kaplan, E. L. 1980. The group A streptococcal upper respiratory tract carrier state: an enigma. *J Pediat* 97:337.

19. Tompkins, R. K., D. C. Burnes, and W. E. Cable. 1977. An analysis of the cost-effectiveness of pharyngitis management and acute rheumatic fever prevention. *Ann Int Med* 86:481.

20. Pantell, R. H. 1981. Pharyngitis: diagnosis and management. *Pediatrics in Review* 3:35.

# 2

# Changing Risk of Rheumatic Fever

## Leon Gordis, M.D., Dr. P.H.

Rheumatic fever has fascinated clinicians and investigators over the years for a variety of reasons. These include the difficulties in its diagnosis, the enigmatic patterns of its natural history, and the etiologic dilemmas that still remain despite the clear implication of the group A beta-hemolytic streptococcus in its causation. These etiologic dilemmas reflect both our inadequate understanding of the pathogenic mechanisms linking the streptococcus to rheumatic fever and the absence of an adequate animal model of the disease. The puzzles remain despite intensive and extensive laboratory investigations of the streptococcus. For despite the organism's almost total loss of privacy and confidentiality, its link to the development of rheumatic fever remains a mystery.

At least part of the fascination of rheumatic fever lies in the fact that it demonstrates that, occasionally, effective prevention may be feasible even in the absence of a good understanding of pathogenic mechanisms linking the putative etiologic agent and the disease. Thus, for example, Jenner was able to develop a prevention for smallpox on the basis of observational data that milkmaids who had developed cowpox were apparently immune when subsequently exposed to smallpox. In the case of rheumatic fever, the streptococcus has been implicated by very different types of evidence—clinical, epidemiologic, and laboratory in nature—and this has provided the basis for prevention, both primary and secondary. In light of these approaches, which have been practiced in the United States to varying degrees for almost 40 years, it is worth examining the patterns of change in risk of rheumatic fever over this time and addressing the implications of these observations for our current approaches for the prevention of rheumatic fever, and specifically, to the diagnosis and treatment of pharyngitis.

In order to assess the extent of changes in rates of rheumatic fever, we can look at mortality or morbidity and focus on rheumatic fever or on rheumatic heart disease. Figure 2–1 shows the trends over time in mortality from acute rheumatic fever and rheumatic heart disease in the United States from 1940 to 1977. A clear decline in deaths from rheumatic fever has taken place since 1940; in recent years the rate has remained extremely low. Mortality from rheumatic heart disease has also declined markedly over this time, although not to the same extent as that from rheumatic fever. We are, of course, dealing with different cohorts, so that the impact of preventing rheumatic fever in one "generation" might not yet be evidenced by reduced mortality from rheumatic heart disease in the other. Above and beyond this problem, we recognize that mortality is a poor index of change in risk of rheumatic fever and rheumatic heart disease because the major long-term impact of rheumatic fever is likely to be disabling rheumatic heart disease rather than mortality.

Figure 2–1. Crude U.S. Death Rates for RF and RHD, 1940–77 (Races and Sexes Combined, All Ages)

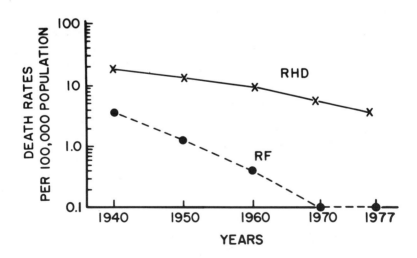

In seeking some measure of the changing risk of rheumatic fever, we clearly wish to estimate changes in the *incidence* of rheumatic fever over time. Over the past fifteen years, we have conducted a series of studies in Baltimore of the changing patterns of rheumatic fever that I should like to review as a basis for our discussion.

Our studies began in the late 1960s. At that time we carried out a review of hospital records in Baltimore in order to use hospital admissions for rheumatic fever to estimate its incidence in residents of the Baltimore metropolitan area [1]. Since it was recognized that some children who are diagnosed by their physicians as having rheumatic fever may not be hospitalized, a telephone survey of physicians was also carried out over a three-month period to determine the proportion of children with rheumatic fever who were not hospitalized. Some results of this initial study covering the years 1960 to 1964, are seen in Table 2–1.

TABLE 2-1. Incidence Rates of Hospitalized Cases of Rheumatic Fever, Ages 5-19, Baltimore, 1960-64

|  | Annual incidence per 100,000 | | |
|---|---|---|---|
|  | First attacks | Recurrences | Total |
| Whites | 8.6 | 1.0 | 9.6 |
| Blacks | 20.2 | 4.2 | 24.4 |
| Total | 13.3 | 2.3 | 15.6 |

In the next few years, it was widely felt that rheumatic fever admission rates were declining in Baltimore, as well as elsewhere in the United States. In order to explore this possibility, a follow-up study was carried out for the years 1968–70, duplicating as much as possible the methodology employed in the first study so that the results of this follow-up could be compared with the initial study [2].

The most dramatic finding in this study was the decline of rheumatic fever in blacks (Table 2–2). While in the early period 1960–64, the rate of rheumatic fever in blacks was 2.5 times the white rate for initial attacks, and 4 times the white rate for recurrences, by 1968–71 the black rate had declined to approximately the same rate seen in whites. The possible reason for these changes will be discussed in a few moments.

TABLE 2-2. Average Annual Incidence Rates of First Attacks of Rheumatic Fever, Ages 5-19, Baltimore, 1960-70

|  | 1960-64 | | 1968-70 | |
|---|---|---|---|---|
|  | No. Cases | Rate | No. Cases | Rate |
| Whites | 61 | 8.6 | 31 | 9.5 |
| Blacks | 98 | 20.2 | 48 | 10.8 |
| Both Races | 159 | 13.3 | 79 | 10.2 |

In recent years, there has been an impression that the risk of rheumatic fever has declined even further. In order to clarify the current picture and to generate comparative data along the lines of our previous studies, we recently initiated a third study of the incidence of rheumatic fever in Baltimore covering the years 1977 to 1981. This study was carried out in virtually the same fashion as the previous two investigations. In order to generate time-trend curves for acute glomerulonephritis (AGN) and to compare them with the time-trend curves for rheumatic fever, data were also collected on AGN for the entire period during which rheumatic fever has been studied—1960 to 1981. The nephritis data are still being analyzed. The results indicate that for first attacks of rheumatic fever, incidence rates have dropped markedly to approximately 0.5 per 100,000 children ages 5–19 for both whites and blacks.

What can account for these dramatic changes? Disease has classically been viewed from the epidemiologic standpoint as the result of an interaction of host, agent, and environment. In looking at the time-trends in incidence of any disease, it is clear that any changes—either up or down—that occur over a relatively short time interval, such as a few decades, cannot be due to changes in the host. The genetic makeup of human populations does not change so quickly. It is therefore necessary to look at changes in the agent and in environmental factors in order to try to explain the sharp decline in incidence and the marked changes in clinical picture and natural history that have occurred in the United States. One possibility is that changes have taken place in the organism itself. We know that changes do occur in endemic and epidemic strains of organisms. Over the past few years, the group B streptococcus has emerged as a major clinical problem—either having been previously less important (less prevalent or of lower virulence) or previously not well recognized. Evidence for a possible change in the organism in the case of the group A streptococcus stems from several observations. Scarlet fever has changed, clearly in severity, and perhaps in incidence as well. In addition, there is suggestive evidence that the incidence of acute poststreptococcal glomerulonephritis has also declined over time.

If a change has indeed occurred in the organism, what might have produced it? What environmental factor could have led to a change in the virulence of the group A streptococcus during this time? An obvious candidate is penicillin. We might speculate that the widespread use of penicillin in the United States has resulted in a high point-prevalence of serum penicillin in American communities at any point in time. This could have served to interrupt the chain of transmission of the streptococcus and to prevent any enhancement of its virulence.

To what extent can we attribute the decline in rheumatic fever to the rational management of streptococcal infections by physicians, a result of intensive programs of physician education, many of which have been carried out over the past several decades? This question was, in fact, examined in a study we conducted in Baltimore several years ago. From 1966 to 1968, a number of comprehensive care programs were established in the inner city of Baltimore. Eligibility for each of these programs was based on census tract of residence. Four of these programs covered contiguous areas in the central city. The rationale of the study was as follows: If the comprehensive care programs were providing quality ambulatory care to the children under their care, this should have included proper treatment of streptococcal infections and should have led to a lower rate of rheumatic fever in children eligible for comprehensive care than in noneligible children.

The city was divided into three areas: a center-city cluster of census tracts eligible for comprehensive care, adjacent noneligible tracts whose residents nevertheless obtained occasional care from the comprehensive care programs because of their close geographic proximity, and finally, nonadjacent, noneligible tracts. The findings are seen in Figures 2–2, 2–3, and 2–4 and strongly suggest the association of a decline in rheumatic fever with eligibility for comprehensive care.

Figure 2–2. Hospitalized First Attacks of Rheumatic Fever, Ages 5–14, Black Population, Baltimore, by Eligibility for Comprehensive Care, 1968–70

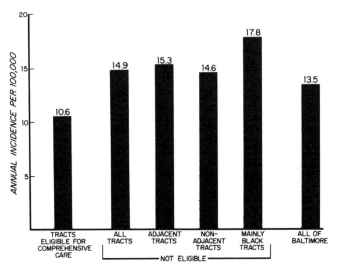

Figure 2–3. Comprehensive Care and Changes in Rheumatic Fever Incidence, Black Population, Ages 5–14, Baltimore, 1960–64 to 1968–70

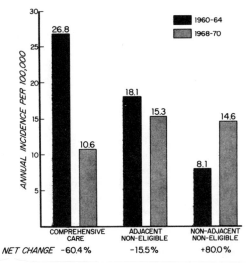

Figure 2–4. Comprehensive Care and Changes in Rheumatic Fever Incidence, Black Population, Ages 5–14, 1960–64 to 1968–70

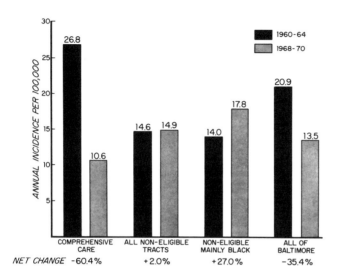

Thus, it seemed clear that rheumatic fever rates had declined selectively in census tracts eligible for comprehensive care. However, it was known that over the years of the study, many social and economic factors had changed in Baltimore aside from the pattern of medical care. Could the decline in rheumatic fever truly be ascribed to the ambulatory care available to these children? In order to answer this question, a further analysis was carried out. If indeed the medical care was responsible for the decline, we would expect the decline to be confined to those children whose cases were preceded by a clinical sore throat and who would therefore have had some reason for consulting their physicians. On the other hand, one would expect no change in rates of rheumatic fever that were not preceded by pharyngitis since these children would not have had any reason to have consulted a physician and thus there would have been no opportunity for primary prevention. The findings from this analysis are consistent with the conclusion that the decline in rheumatic fever in Baltimore during this time was due primarily to the comprehensive care programs or to some very closely related factor.

It is of interest, I believe, to ask whether comprehensive care could indeed have had such an effect in view of the known high levels of noncompliance in children for whom penicillin is prescribed for pharyngitis. This question is difficult to answer, but it raises the issue whether after only five days of penicillin, the risk of rheumatic fever may be reduced, albeit not to the same level that would be reached after ten days of therapy. Perhaps this should enter our cost-benefit calculations in discussing the most appropriate approach to managing acute pharyngitis today.

An interesting observation made during our recent study in Baltimore is that a large proportion of children discharged from the hospital with the diagnosis of acute rheumatic fever do not seem to meet the revised Jones Criteria [3]. It has long been recognized that the Jones Criteria are less adequate for mild cases of rheumatic fever than for moderate and severe cases. With the apparent change in clinical severity of rheumatic fever in recent years, with most cases being of a mild nature, the Jones Criteria seem less useful. In addition, what has always been a "weak link" in the Jones Criteria, the combination of arthritis, fever, and elevated sedimentation rate, continues to haunt us in the diagnosis of rheumatic fever. Do we have to pursue a different approach for the diagnosis of rheumatic fever in the United States in this era? Another issue raised by our observations is the possibility that many children who would previously have been diagnosed as having rheumatic fever are now diagnosed as having other conditions, such as juvenile rheumatoid arthritis. As diagnostic tools for other illnesses have improved over the years, there has probably been a tendency to classify children who might have previously been diagnosed with rheumatic fever in these new diagnostic categories.

Thus, it seems clear that over the past 20 years in Baltimore there has been a marked decline in the incidence of rheumatic fever, bordering on virtual disappearance of the disease. The factors that have contributed to this remain unclear. Although comprehensive care programs appear to have been a major factor in the decline from 1960–64 to 1968–70, they primarily led to a decrease in rates among blacks which became comparable to the rates of whites. From 1968–70 to 1977–81, however, a dramatic decline took place in rheumatic fever rates in both whites and blacks, a change that is difficult to account for by any single factor.

Our data deal with the incidence of rheumatic fever in the general population, rather than the incidence of rheumatic fever in those who have had a streptococcal infection. The latter information would be of great value, but unfortunately is not available. Nor are data available regarding the changing incidence of streptococcal infections, particularly of streptococcal pharyngitis. Thus at the present time, we do not have the data base needed to estimate the risk of rheumatic fever associated with a streptococcal infection.

Nevertheless, the extraordinarily low rates of rheumatic fever and the mildness of the disease seen recently in Baltimore suggest that the risk is extremely low. If the Baltimore data are characteristic of other cities in the United States as well, the low rates raise the question of whether a more relaxed policy regarding the diagnosis and treatment of pharyngitis may be warranted. In considering such a policy, however, we must consider the possibility that the current state of affairs—that is, the low rates of rheumatic fever seen today—may have resulted from the strong policy regarding pharyngitis that was pursued for many years, and whether relaxation of this policy might lead to a resurgence of the high risk of rheumatic fever with the severe clinical picture seen so frequently several decades ago.

Just how much of the bright picture we see today is attributable to rigorous medical approaches to diagnosis and treatment and how much to other unplanned and perhaps as yet unidentified changes in our urban environment remains unclear. Are we perhaps witnessing a situation such as we have seen for traffic accidents? As Etzioni pointed out [4], a variety of driver educational programs and programs addressing the danger of the automobile itself for many years failed to affect the increasing rate of traffic fatalities and injuries. What these organized and directed efforts failed to accomplish, however, was achieved by imposition of the 55-mile-per-hour speed limit in response to the energy crisis: a marked reduction in the number of traffic deaths per year. Thus, an unforeseen change, occurring for different reasons or introduced for an entirely different purpose, may succeed in doing what numerous directed efforts at prevention may not accomplish.

## REFERENCES

1. Gordis L, A. Lilienfeld, and R. Rodriguez. 1969. Studies in the epidemiology and preventability of rheumatic fever—I. demographic factors and the incidence of acute attacks. *J Chron Dis* 21:645–854.

2. Gordis L. 1973. Effectiveness of comprehensive-care programs in preventing rheumatic fever. *New Engl J Med* 289:331–35.

3. American Heart Association. 1965. Jones Criteria (revised) for guidance in the diagnosis of rheumatic fever. *Circulation* 32:664.

4. Etzioni A. 1974. The humility factor. *Science* 185:4154.

# 3

# Incidence of Acute Rheumatic Fever in Memphis and Shelby County, Tennessee, 1977-81

*Alan L. Bisno, M.D.,*
*and Mack A. Land, M.D.*

Development of rational strategies for management of streptococcal pharyngitis at present and in the near future depends, in good measure, upon precise knowledge of the incidence of acute rheumatic fever (ARF). There is ample evidence that this incidence has declined markedly over the past 50 years in North America and western Europe [1]. Detailed data on the incidence of ARF in urban areas in the United States, however, are quite limited. The well-known studies conducted in Baltimore [2], Nashville [3], and the borough of Manhattan [4] were all completed during the 1960s, well over a decade ago. We therefore undertook a survey of ARF incidence for the years 1977–81, inclusive, in a major urban population center of the southeastern United States, Memphis and Shelby County, Tennessee.

We reviewed the hospital records of all patients discharged with a diagnosis of ARF or Sydenham's chorea from 12 of the 13 general medical-surgical hospitals in Memphis-Shelby County for the study period. Diagnoses reviewed included the following categories listed in the International Classification of Diseases: 390, rheumatic fever without mention of heart involvement; 391, rheumatic fever with heart involvement; and 392, rheumatic chorea. One

This work was supported in part by Grant No. AI-10085 from the National Institutes of Health and Grant No. 80–981 from the American Heart Association.

hospital, a 243-bed community medical-surgical hospital, was unable to furnish the information requested. Records of the Rheumatic Fever Research Project, a program in existence since 1965, were also reviewed to identify primary or recurrent cases missed by hospital chart reviews. In addition, 327 family practitioners, internists (including cardiologists and rheumatologists), pediatricians, and neurologists in Memphis-Shelby County were surveyed by mail to determine whether they had identified any cases of ARF during the study period. Those who failed to return the stamped, self-addressed reply card or those who responded affirmatively were contacted by telephone to obtain necessary information.

Cases were included in this study only if they fulfilled the modified Jones Criteria [5]. Race, sex, and age-specific population figures for Memphis-Shelby County, as well as economic data relative to respective census tracts, were those of the 1980 U.S. census. Statistical comparisons of incidence rates were determined by the method of testing equality of two percentages [6].

We identified 56 cases diagnosed as ARF during the five-year study period. No individual had more than one attack. Fifteen cases were omitted from further consideration because they failed to meet the modified Jones criteria. Of the remaining 41 cases accepted as genuine, 34 were first attacks and seven (17%) were recurrences. Twenty-five of the 41 patients were residents of Memphis-Shelby County. The 16 who resided outside the county were not included in analyses of attack rates but were considered in tabulations of clinical manifestations.

The overall incidence of ARF in Memphis-Shelby County for 1977–81 was 0.64 cases/100,000 population/year (Table 3–1). The age range was 3 to 57 years. As expected, the peak age incidence (1.88/100,000 population/year) was in the 5–17 year age group. The disease was much more common in blacks than whites (Table 3–2), and the incidence rates for the two races differed significantly in both the 5–17 ($p = 0.01$) and 18–64 ($p < 0.01$) age groups.

Sixty percent of ARF cases occurred in inner city census tracts (Figure 3–1), which are populated predominantly by Memphians who are both poor and black. For example, considering inner city tracts in which a case of ARF occurred, the average black population aged 5–17 years was 1509, while the average white population was 43. The average of the median values for housing in these same tracts was $24,572. The boundaries we selected to define the "inner city" were, however, arbitrary and contain within them areas of widely varying socioeconomic status.

TABLE 3-1.  Incidence of ARF by Age Group in Memphis-Shelby County, Tennessee, 1977-81

| Age group (years) | No. of patients | Population at risk | Incidence (cases/100,000 population/year) |
|---|---|---|---|
| < 5 | 1 | 60,736 | 0.33 |
| 5-17 | 16 | 169,935 | 1.88 |
| 18-64 | 8 | 473,564 | 0.34 |
| ≧ 65 | 0 | 72,878 | 0 |
| Total | 25 | 777,113 | 0.64 |

Source: Reprinted from Land, M. A., and A. L. Bisno. 1983. _JAMA_ 249-895 (with permission).

TABLE 3-2.  Incidence of ARF by Race and Age Group Memphis-Shelby County, Tennessee, 1977-81

| Race | Age group (years) | | | |
|---|---|---|---|---|
| | < 5 | 5-17 | 18-64 | ≧ 65 |
| **Black** | | | | |
| No. cases | 1 | 12 | 7 | 0 |
| Population | 31,826 | 89,306 | 176,163 | 27,369 |
| Incidence* | 0.63 | 2.69 | 0.79 | 0 |
| **White** | | | | |
| No. cases | 0 | 3 | 1 | 0 |
| Population | 28,173 | 79,180 | 292,826 | 45,279 |
| Incidence* | 0 | 0.76 | 0.07 | 0 |
| **Other** | | | | |
| No. cases | 0 | 1† | 0 | 0 |
| Population | 737 | 1,449 | 4,575 | 230 |
| Incidence* | 0 | 13.8 | 0 | 0 |

*Cases/100,000 population/year.
†This case occurred in an Oriental girl.
Source: Reprinted from Land, M. A., and A. L. Bisno. 1983. _JAMA_ 249:895 (with permission).

Figure 3–1. Location, by census tract, of residences of patients with ARF. Short bold dashes indicate inner city. Long thin dashes indicate city limits.

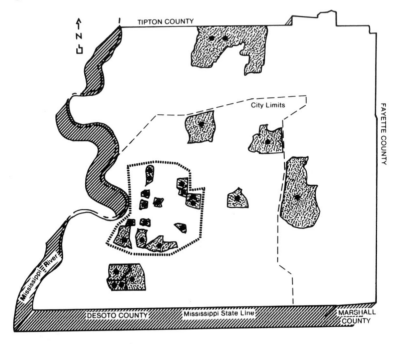

Reprinted from Land, M. A., and A. L. Bisno. 1983. *JAMA* 249:895 (with permission).

The ARF incidence was 2.7-fold higher in black school children residing in the inner city than among black sub-urbanites. A similar trend was discernible for whites, but the numbers of cases were very small (Figure 3–2). The incidence of ARF among white school children residing outside the inner city has fallen to strikingly low levels—approximately one case per 200,000 children per year.

The distribution of clinical manifestations of ARF was similar in the 25 Memphis-Shelby County residents and the 16 patients from surrounding areas; the two groups have therefore been combined. The most common major manifestation was polyarthritis, which was present in 61% of patients, followed by carditis (54%), chorea (27%), and erythema marginatum (10%). Subcutaneous nodules were noted in only one case (2%). Five of the 22 patients with carditis suffered congestive heart failure; this represents 12% of the total group of 41 ARF patients. Twenty-eight

Figure 3–2. Incidence of ARF by race and area of residence for 5 to 17-year old children, Memphis and Shelby County, Tennessee, 1977–81

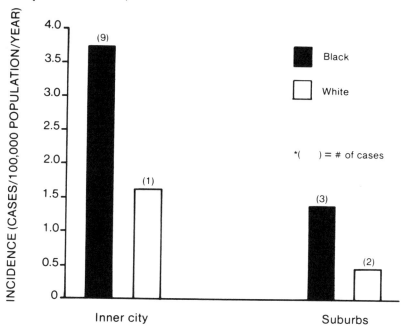

patients (68%) gave a history of preceding upper respiratory infection or sore throat in the four weeks prior to onset of symptoms of ARF. The seasonal distribution of cases was winter, 40%; spring, 28%; summer, 8%; fall, 24%.

The ARF incidence reported here is the lowest ever recorded for a major U.S. metropolitan area. The urban studies conducted during the 1960s [2,3,4] yielded estimated ARF attack rates among school children ranging from 24 to 61 per 100,000 (Figure 3–3). A recent report from a smaller community, Rochester, Minnesota [7], indicated an ARF rate of 9 per 100,000 among 5 to 14-year old children between 1965 and 1978. Recent data from statewide surveys [8,9,10,11,12] and from the Navajo Indian reservation [13] in the desert Southwest are summarized in Table 3–3. Even in these settings, which are partially or totally non-urban, the rates exceed our current Memphis incidence. Interestingly, the data most comparable to our own were collected several years ago from our neighboring state of Mississippi (Table 3–3) [9].

Are the extraordinarily low ARF rates reported here the result of methodologic errors? It is unlikely that appreciable numbers of ARF cases occurring in Memphis residents

Figure 3–3. Comparative incidence of ARF in school-aged children in various urban centers, 1960–81

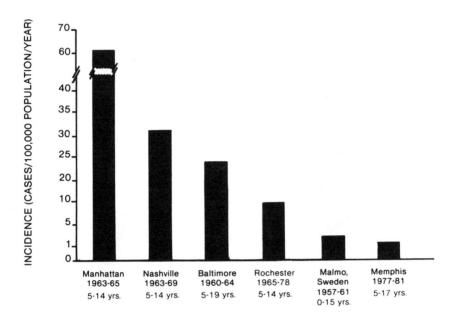

were diagnosed and treated elsewhere, because there are no major metropolitan centers within a 100-mile radius of the city. Within the city, we reviewed diligently the records of the 12 major public and private general hospitals. The one general hospital unable to provide us with discharge diagnoses has less than 2% of all beds in the county and has no pediatric or indigent services. The long-standing interest of our investigative group in ARF is well-known in the community, and thus cases are frequently called to our attention by attending physicians or housestaff either by receipt of throat swabs and serologic specimens in our research lab or by requests for clinical consultation.

We endeavored to identify nonhospitalized cases by personal solicitation of case reports from practitioners judged likely to see patients with ARF. Indeed, a number of the 41 cases we ultimately identified were reported by this method. All were hospitalized cases also identified by our chart review, however. Two nonhospitalized cases were omitted, because, on review of office files, the diagnoses were judged too tenuous for inclusion.

The fact that we were unable to identify any nonhospitalized patients suggests our retrospective attempts at

TABLE 3-3.  Incidence of ARF during 1960s and 1970s in Various Populations*

| Locale | Year | Ref. | Age group (yrs.) | Incidence (100,000 pop./yr.) | Remarks |
|--------|------|------|------------------|------------------------------|---------|
| Missouri | 1979 | 8 | All ages | 4.95 | Hospitalized and |
|  |  |  | 5-9 | 12.90 | nonhospitalized |
|  |  |  | 10-14 | 12.75 | cases |
| Mississippi | 1964-73 | 9 | All ages | 1.9 | Hospitalized cases |
|  |  |  | 10-14 | 6.2 | only |
| Connecticut | 1968-72 | 10 | All ages | 2.9 | Hospitalized cases only |
| Oklahoma | 1969 | 11 | All ages | 4.2 | Hospitalized cases |
|  |  |  | 5-9 | 11.3 | only |
|  |  |  | 10-14 | 14.2 |  |
| Colorado | 1973 | 12 | All ages | 5.9 | Rough approximation from reports by a physician panel |
| Navajo Reservation (Ariz., N. Mex., Utah) | 1974-75 1972-77 | 13 | All ages 5-24 | 11.2 13.4 | Hospitalized cases only. Incidence in 5-24-year age group includes only initial attacks |

*For data on surveys conducted in exclusively urban settings, see Figure 3-3.

physician reporting may well have been inadequate.  Surveys in Baltimore [2] and in Missouri [8] found approximately 36% and 47%, respectively, of the total number of ARF cases to have been managed as outpatients.  Even allowing for an error of this magnitude, which seems unlikely in the Memphis setting, the ARF rates in Memphis-Shelby County for 1977–81 are remarkably low.  There is precedent for the extremely low urban ARF incidence reported here, but not in the United States.  Workers in Copenhagen, Denmark, and Malmö, Sweden, [14] found that, by the early 1960s, ARF incidence had plummeted to approximately 1.5/100,000 with rates in Swedish children (less than 16 years of age) being 2.3/100,000 [15].

When ARF does occur in Memphis, it continues to be a disease of indigent black children and young adults. The ratio of black-to-white cases was 5:1. The disease has become extremely rare in the more affluent, largely white suburbs.

We do not have precise data on the incidence of ARF in Memphis in the years preceding 1977. As elsewhere in the U.S., however, it has declined precipitously. In the late 1960s and early 1970s, for example, ten to 26 ARF cases were admitted each year to City of Memphis Hospital alone [16,17]. The reasons for the abrupt decline are incompletely understood. Multiple factors are likely involved, include improved living standards with decreased crowding, antimicrobial therapy for primary and secondary ARF prevention, and decline in rheumatogenic potential of currently prevalent group A streptococcal strains [16,17,18].

Historically the southeastern United States has been an area of relatively low ARF incidence [19]. It remains to be seen whether ARF attack rates have declined to this remarkable extent in the suburbs of cities in other geographic regions of the country. If so, this fact must be taken into account in formulating future strategies for prevention of rheumatic fever. Issues such as the necessity for identifying treatment failures, the importance of culturing household contacts, the advisability of using benzathine penicillin G for primary prevention of ARF, and the duration of secondary prophylaxis must all be reassessed in view of the extreme rarity of the disease in populations served by private primary care practitioners.

## REFERENCES

1. Stollerman, G. H. 1975. *Rheumatic Fever and Streptococcal Infection,* 63–100. New York: Grune and Stratton.

2. Gordis, L., A. Lilienfeld, and R. Rodriguez. 1969. Studies in the epidemiology and preventability of rheumatic fever—I: demographic factors and the incidence of acute attacks. *J Chron Dis* 21:645.

3. Quinn, R. W., and C. F. Federspiel. 1974. The incidence of rheumatic fever in metropolitan Nashville, 1963–1969. *Amer J Epidemiol* 99:273.

4. Brownell, K. D., and F. Bailen-Rose. 1973. Acute rheumatic fever in children: incidence in a borough of New York City. *JAMA* 224:1593.

5. American Heart Association. 1965. Jones criteria (revised) for guidance in the diagnosis of rheumatic fever. *Circ* 32:664.

6. Sokel, R. R., and F. J. Rolhf. 1969. *Biometry,* 607–8. San Francisco: W. H. Freeman.

7. Annegers, J. F., N. L. Pillman, W. H. Weidman et al. 1982. Rheumatic fever in Minnesota, 1935–1978. *Mayo Clin Proc* 57:753.

8. Allen, W. C. 1982. Rheumatic fever and rheumatic heart disease in Missouri. *Missouri Med* 29:219.

9. Powell, K. E., and D. G. Watson. 1981. Acute rheumatic fever in Mississippi: a survey of hospitalized cases, 1964 to 1973. *So Med J* 74:553.

10. Markowitz, M. 1977. The changing picture of rheumatic fever. *Arth Rheum* 20:369.

11. Silberg, S. L., S. W. Ferguson, and P. S. Anderson. 1971. Incidence of acute rheumatic fever and rheumatic heart disease in Oklahoma. *J Okla Med Assoc* 64:477.

12. Rhodes, P., and H. Jackson. 1975. Rheumatic fever in Colorado: a conquered disease? *JAMA* 234:157.

13. Coulehan, J., S. Grant, K. Reisinger et al. 1980. Acute rheumatic fever and rheumatic heart disease on the Navajo Reservation. *Publ Hlth Rep* 95:62.

14. Sievers, J., and P. Hall. 1971. Incidence of acute rheumatic fever. *Brit Heart J* 33:833.

15. Ekelund, H., E. Enocksson, M. Michaelsson et al. 1967. The incidence of acute rheumatic fever in Swedish children 1952–61. A survey from four hospitals. *Acta Med Scand* 181:89.

16. Bisno, A. L., I. A. Pearce, H. P. Wall et al. 1970. Contrasting epidemiology of acute rheumatic fever and acute glomerulonephritis: nature of the antecendent streptococcal infection. *New Engl J Med* 283:561.

17. Bisno, A. L. 1980. The concept of rheumatogenic and non-rheumatogenic group A streptococci. In *Streptococcal Diseases and the Immune Response* 136:278. S. E. Read, and J. B. Zabriskie, ed. New York: Academic Press.

18. Bisno, A. L., I. A. Pearce, and G. H. Stollerman. 1977. Streptococcal infections that fail to cause recurrences of rheumatic fever. *J Infec Dis* 136:278.

19. Schwentker, F. F. 1952. The epidemiology of rheumatic fever. In *Rheumatic Fever: A symposium*. L. Thomas, ed. Minneapolis: University of Minnesota Press.

# 4

# Diagnosis of Pharyngitis: Clinical and Epidemiologic Features

*Lewis W. Wannamaker, M.D.*

Basic to any discriminative plan for the management of pharyngitis is the question of how to assure an accurate etiologic diagnosis. Physicians differ widely in the confidence they hold in their clinical ability to distinguish between streptococcal and nonstreptococcal infections of the upper respiratory tract, in the reliability they place in throat cultures, and in their opinions concerning the need to make a distinction [1]. I will assume in this discussion that there is an advantage in making a differentiation. Whether this benefit is health effective, cost effective, or merely intellectually satisfying in the United States at the present time is the crux of the issues that we are wrestling with at this conference.

There is general agreement about the classical features of streptococcal pharyngitis (Table 4-1). The rub is that many streptococcal infections do not exhibit the classical features of streptococcal pharyngitis and that other infectious agents can mimic streptococcal infections.

Many attempts have been made to define streptococcal infections. Considering the differences in these studies, it is not surprising that consensus on a universal approach to diagnosis is difficult to reach. These studies have varied in the population groups chosen for study, in criteria for admission to the study, in the conditions for exclusion from the study, and finally in the criteria used for final confirmation or definition of infection.

TABLE 4-1.  Classical Features of Streptococcal Pharyngitis

---

Sudden onset
Sore throat (pain on swallowing)
Fever
Headache
Nausea, vomiting, abdominal pain
  (especially in children)
Marked inflammation of throat and tonsils
Patchy discrete exudate
Tender, enlarged anterior cervical nodes

Rare (suggestive of other etiologies):

Conjunctivitis, cough, diarrhea
Nasal discharge (except in young children)

---

Population groups have included children [2-10] or adults [11-14] (or both [15-18]), civilian [2-10,14-18], or military personnel [11-13], private or group practice [2,3,5,6,9,10,15], ambulatory clinic [4,14] or emergency room [8] patients, and families (either rheumatic [7,16,18] or nonrheumatic [6,16,18]). Criteria for admission to a study have shown a wide range. Some have been broadly inclusive, embracing any respiratory or febrile illness [7]. Others have admitted all acute respiratory infections [3,10] or all upper respiratory infections [5]. Still others have included only patients with symptoms or signs of sore throat [4,6,8,9,14,15], and some have required an unsolicited complaint of sore throat [17]. Still more restrictive are studies that have focused on patients with exudative tonsillitis or pharyngitis [11-13]. Some have been rather indefinite in their criteria for admission, including any patient who "might have streptococcal infection" [2]. A number of studies have had specified exclusions, such as suppurative complications [8], profuse serous nasal secretions [15], frequent cough [15], or prior antibiotic treatment [4,5,17].

The criterion used as confirming evidence of streptococcal infection has almost always been based on the results of throat cultures. Some studies have accepted or analyzed for all beta-hemolytic streptococci [2–5,8–13,15,16,18]. Others have been limited to or have also analyzed for group A streptococci [4,6–8,11–18]. Some have required a minimum number of beta-hemolytic colonies on the culture plate [10], usually ten or more, sometimes 50 or more

colonies. Some have focused on acquisition of beta-hemolytic or group A streptococci, with or without evidence of
clinical disease [16,18]. Relatively few studies have used
streptococcal antibodies for the definition of infection.
Some have used ASO [7,11–13], others multiple antibodies
[4,8,15,16]. A prompt clinical response after initiation of
antibiotic therapy has been viewed as further evidence of
streptococcal infection by some physicians, but this may be
somewhat specious in differentiating between acute respiratory illnesses, many of which last only a few days regardless of whether they are bacterial or nonbacterial and
whether or not they are treated with antibiotics.

In addition to these variables in the design of studies,
epidemiologic factors may have a profound influence on the
accuracy of diagnosis of streptococcal upper respiratory
infections (Table 4–2). In an epidemic situation, once the
agent is identified, the accuracy is often close to 100% even
in cases with borderline manifestations. During a food-
borne outbreak, physicians may develop an exhilarating
confidence in their diagnostic perspicacity, resulting from
the sudden appearance of a large number of cases with
remarkably uniform classical manifestations. This exag-
gerated self-confidence may be rapidly deflated when dealing with the much more common problem of endemic infections in children, of whom a number may be experiencing
incomplete or atypical manifestations of streptococcal infection against a background of multiple respiratory agents
and a high streptococcal carrier rate. In some populations,
carrier rates build up to high levels—sometimes exceeding
50%—towards the end of the streptococcal respiratory
season. The introduction of a nonstreptococcal pharyn-
gitis-producing agent into such a population may result in a
large number of misguided diagnoses. In patients with
pharyngitis and a positive throat culture, the presence of a
high acute phase streptococcal antibody test enhances the
possibility that the patient is a carrier rather than one with
active streptococcal infection [8]. We are rarely if ever
operating in a vacuum of no other respiratory illnesses and
no chronic carriers of beta-hemolytic streptococci.

Other factors or findings may increase the diagnostic
accuracy of streptococcal infection of the upper respiratory
tract. There may be a history of close contact with a
well-documented case of streptococcal infection, an often
neglected but valuable clue. Physical signs that are almost
pathognomonic include, of course, the rash and other
manifestations of scarlet fever. Excoriated nares, mostly
found in infants, are also strongly indicative of streptococcal infection, as are "doughnut" lesions on the palate,

TABLE 4-2.  Epidemiologic Factors Influencing the Accuracy of Diagnosis

| Enhancing factors | Diminishing factors |
| --- | --- |
| Epidemic (that is, food-borne) | Endemic situation |
| Absence of other respiratory agents | Multiple respiratory agents |
| Low carrier rate | High carrier rate |
| Older population | Younger population |
| Low acute phase antibody titers | High acute phase antibody titers |

often mistaken for petechiae but clearly described by Amren [19] (Figure 4–1). True petechiae of the throat or palate are occasionally present but may be found in other illnesses. Unfortunately, all of these highly suggestive physical signs are found in only a small fraction of patients.

Figure 4–1. "Doughnut" lesions on the palate, strongly indicative of streptococcal infection.

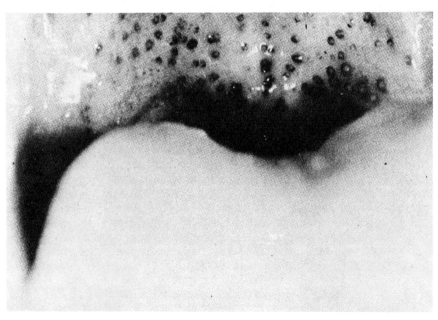

(From Breese [20].)
*Note*: The pale centers may be smaller and less obvious [19] than depicted here.

The presence of tonsils may facilitate the visibility of exudate. Diagnosis is more accurate when the patient presents at the time the clinical picture is fullblown. The studies of Breese and Disney [2] have demonstrated that clinical discrimination of streptococcal from nonstreptococcal illness is less reliable when the patient is seen less than 12 hours or more than four days after onset of illness (Figure 4–2).

Figure 4–2. Relationship of time seen after onset of illness to accuracy of clinical diagnosis.

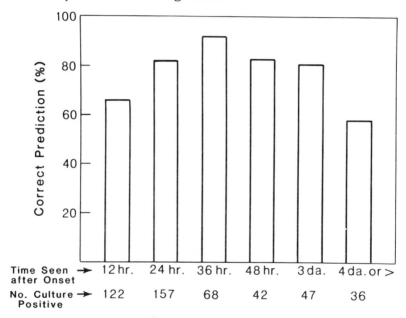

(Modified from Breese and Disney [2].)

The use of white blood cell counts as a means of differentiating streptococcal from nonstreptococcal pharyngitis is viewed with varying enthusiasm. They seem to be more helpful in adults than in children who more frequently respond to viral infection with an increase in white blood cell count. The studies of Breese and Disney in children (Figure 4–3) show a difference in distribution of counts between streptococcal and nonstreptococcal illnesses, but the distinction is not clear cut. The differentiation appears to be most dependable in children with white blood cell counts of less than 12,500 mm$^3$; these children are unlikely to have a positive throat culture for beta-hemolytic streptococci.

Figure 4–3. Distribution of white blood cell counts in culture-positive and culture-negative patients

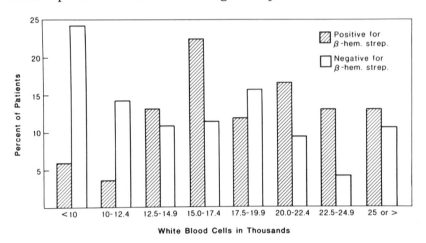

(Modified from Breese and Disney [2].)

The effect of the age of the patient on the accuracy of diagnosis of streptococcal upper respiratory infection was well documented in the studies of Breese and Disney [2] who found that the percentage of correct prediction of culture results from clinical findings was significantly less in infants than in older children (Figure 4–4). As with older children, it appears from the studies of Walsh and coworkers [14] that clinical differentiation of streptococcal from nonstreptococcal upper respiratory infection in adults is generally more reliable than in younger age groups.

The clinical picture in children under three years of age was well described in the classic studies of Powers and Boisvert [21] who called this subacute, constitutional (rather than localized) form of streptococcal illness "streptococcal fever, childhood type" (Table 4–3).

Other studies have indicated that exudative tonsillitis in children less than three years of age is usually not streptococcal [22]. Currently in the United States, streptococcal infections appear to be relatively uncommon in children under three years of age. By contrast, studies in Egypt, one of many developing countries where rheumatic heart disease is a major problem, indicate that acquisitions of group A streptococci are frequent in infants and preschool children [18]. This finding raises the question of whether acquisition of group A streptococci early in life is a requisite for the development of rheumatic fever. Matanoski and colleagues [16] demonstrated a higher streptococcal

Figure 4–4. Relationship of age to accuracy of clinical diagnosis.

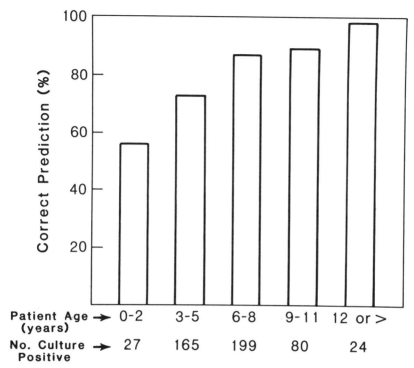

Patient Age → (years): 0-2, 3-5, 6-8, 9-11, 12 or >

No. Culture Positive →: 27, 165, 199, 80, 24

(Modified from Breese and Disney [2].)

TABLE 4-3. Streptococcal Fever, Childhood Type (< 3 yrs.)

Subacute constitutional reaction
Mild rhinopharyngitis
Thin excoriating nasal discharge
Moderate to low grade fever (4-8 wks.)
Moderate cervical adenitis, sometimes suppurative
Catarrhal or suppurative otitis media
Occasional bacteremia
Suppurative complications not infrequent
Nonsuppurative sequelae rare

Source: Powers and Boisvert [21].

infection rate in infants from rheumatic as compared to nonrheumatic families. If infection early in life is a key factor in the pathogenesis of rheumatic fever, the importance of recognition and treatment of streptococcal infections in infants may be greater than we have previously recognized.

We shall now examine the reliability of single findings or combinations of findings in the diagnosis of streptococcal respiratory infections. Of the common findings, rarely can any single one be depended upon. In studies by our Minnesota group, Kaplan and coworkers [8] used antibody responses to streptolysin O and to streptococcal desoxyribonuclease B (DNAse B) in addition to culture results as a means of defining streptococcal infection. In these studies, anterior cervical lymphadenitis was the clinical finding that correlated best with the demonstration of a rise in streptococcal antibodies. Despite the probability of some suppression by antibiotic therapy, 61% of children with group A streptococci and tender anterior cervical nodes showed an antibody response to one or both of these antigens. No other *single* clinical symptom or sign showed a statistically significant difference in frequency of antibody response. As Dr. Kaplan will discuss later in this symposium, this study of antibody responses was designed primarily to differentiate active streptococcal infection from the carrier state in the symptomatic child [8]. This distinction is one of the most difficult problems we face in the diagnosis of streptococcal infections of the upper respiratory tract.

Combinations of findings have been generally more useful than single ones. A long term observer of the streptococcal scene is Maxwell Stillerman. He and his associate, Stanley Bernstein [15], evaluated clinical syndromes in the diagnosis of streptococcal pharyngitis. In their studies, four combinations of findings were strongly predictive of a positive throat culture for beta-hemolytic streptococci (Figure 4–5). These included several but not all combinations of significant pharyngeal redness or edema, exudate, "petechiae" (which apparently included "doughnut" lesions), and adenitis. Unfortunately, these highly suggestive syndromes were found in only 36% of streptococcal cases.

A somewhat different approach was taken by Burtis Breese, an astute appraiser of streptococcal respiratory infections for many years. Breese [3] has devised a scoring system that assigns weights to nine factors he found useful in the differentiation of streptococcal from nonstreptococcal illnesses (Table 4–4). These include two epidemiologic factors (season and age), five clinical factors

Figure 4–5. The predictive value of various clinical syndromes in the diagnosis of streptococcal pharyngitis.

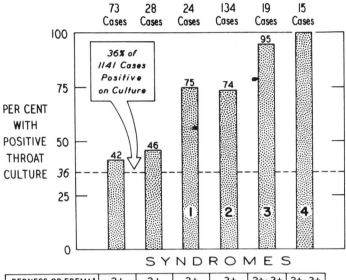

| REDNESS OR EDEMA* | 2+ | 2+ | 2+ | 3+ | 2+-3+ | 2+-3+ |
|---|---|---|---|---|---|---|
| EXUDATE | O | 2+-3+ | 2+-3+ | O -3+ | O | 1+-3+ |
| PETECHIAE | O | O | O | O | 2+-3+ | 1+-3+ |
| ADENITIS** | + | O | + | ± | ± | ± |

*"O" indicates absence; 1+, 2+ or 3+ indicate slight, moderate or marked grades of severity.
** Large tender nodes are indicated by "+", absence by "O" and presence or absence by "±".

(From Stillerman and Bernstein [15].)

TABLE 4-4. Nine Factor Scoring System

---

Season
Age
Fever (≧ 100.5)
Sore throat
Headache
Abnormal pharynx
Abnormal cervical glands
Cough
WBC count

---

Source: Breese [3].

that favor streptococcal infection, one symptom (cough) the presence of which weighs *against* streptococcal infection, and one laboratory determination (WBC count). Children and adolescents with acute respiratory illness were divided into four groups of unequal size in which the culture predictions were negative, maybe negative, maybe positive, and positive on the basis of scores (Figure 4–6). In these studies the percentage of correct prediction was high in the the 20% of patients judged clinically to be culture-negative and in the 44% of patients predicted to be culture-positive. In the two intermediate groups, comprising 36% of patients, culture prediction was less reliable. Clearly, it is this sizeable intermediate group that gives the most trouble if we depend on clinical manifestations (plus white blood cell count). Overall, the culture result was predicted correctly from the clinical score in 77.8% of patients with acute respiratory infections. It is disappointing that the percentage of correct prediction from this clinical scoring system was no better than the tentative diagnosis assigned without the use of the scoring system [3]. This suggests that the scoring system may be useful for some medical providers but may offer no real advantage to experienced observers of streptococcal illnesses. It should also be noted that, despite the generally favorable predictive value of clinical scores and impressions recorded in these studies, Breese is a firm supporter of a throat culture as "the best single practical means of confirming a streptococcal diagnosis" [20].

Figure 4–6. Percentage of correct culture prediction from clinical score in children with acute respiratory disease.

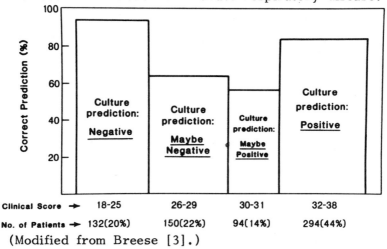

(Modified from Breese [3].)

The success of Breese and his associate, Frank Disney, in predicting culture results from clinical findings is higher than that reported by some other observers, who have found the predictive value of clinical impressions to be closer to 50%. Several factors may have contributed to the favorable results reported by Breese. Breese and Disney are unusually perceptive and experienced students of streptococcal illnesses, no doubt a significant factor. They also had the advantage of constant appraisal of clinical impressions by culture results, which is a powerful means of refining clinical acumen and a valuable indicator of what is currently "going around" in a community. In addition, as part of the clinical evaluation, these investigators had available a white blood cell count, a laboratory test not always obtained or not considered by some an appropriate part of *clinical* predictions.

Results from the private practice population of Breese and Disney may not be applicable to other population groups. For example, clinic populations may differ in the reporting of symptoms and may have higher streptococcal carrier rates than the 5% to 10% found by Breese. As noted earlier, the value of positive throat cultures as confirmation of active streptococcal infection is clearly reduced in populations with high carrier rates [8]. In addition, the percent of correct predictions was probably favored in the studies of Breese [3] by including all patients with acute respiratory infection rather than only those with pharyngitis, since one would expect a high frequency of correct predictions of negative cultures in those without manifestations of pharyngitis, especially with a low background carrier rate. This would tend to boost the overall percent of correct predictions. Clearly, further studies are needed to evaluate the general applicability of this and other scoring systems in different situations, especially in settings other than private practice, for instance, in clinic populations where the risk of rheumatic fever may be higher than in private practice patients.

Before closing, the thorny problem of asymptomatic or subclinical infections should be considered. These are apparently quite common, possibly responsible for spread of infection, and considered to be liable for a significant proportion of patients who develop nonsuppurative complications. Investigators, as well as practicing physicians, find them difficult to detect and to differentiate from the carrier state. In the barrack studies of streptococcal infections at Warren Air Force Base, we found that two-thirds of young adults who acquired and continued to harbor a new serological type of group A streptococcus for at least several weeks were asymptomatic, even though some of them exhibited florid exudative pharyngitis on inspection and most of them developed a rise in ASO titer. Further studies of this problem are needed in civilian populations in different epidemiological settings.

In conclusion, epidemiologic and clinical findings are an essential part of the diagnosis of streptococcal infection of the upper respiratory tract. If streptococcal infections are becoming less severe, as is generally believed, careful and critical documentation of these manifestations may be even more important. In some situations, impressions gained from clinical and epidemiologic findings alone may have a generally good success rate for prediction of culture results. Nevertheless, throat cultures are highly valuable in confirming clinical impressions, in providing a critical appraisal of clinical acumen, and in accurately monitoring the proportion of acute respiratory illnesses due to group A streptococci. The size of the streptococcal slice of the pie varies from population to population and is frequently changing within a population group.

In my view, epidemiologic, clinical, and culture findings are all important. By neglecting any one of them—by necessity or by deliberate choice—we must recognize that we are operating in semi-darkness. At best, the differential diagnosis of streptococcal infection of the upper respiratory tract is an inexact science, one requiring the use and careful evaluation of all available clues and pieces of evidence.

REFERENCES

1. Wannamaker, L. W. 1972. Perplexity and precision in the diagnosis of streptococcal pharyngitis. *Amer J Dis Child* 124:352–58.
2. Breese, B. B., and F. A. Disney. 1954. The accuracy of diagnosis of beta streptococcal infections on clinical grounds. *J Pediatr* 44:670–73.
3. Breese, B. B. 1977. A simple scorecard for the tentative diagnosis of streptococcal pharyngitis. *Am J Dis Child* 131:514–17.
4. Siegel, A. C., E. E. Johnson, and G. H. Stollerman. 1961. Controlled studies of streptococcal pharyngitis in a pediatric population. 1. Factors related to the attack rate of rheumatic fever. *New Engl J Med* 265:559–66.
5. Markowitz, M. 1963. Cultures of the respiratory tract in pediatric practice. *Amer J Dis Child* 105:46–52.
6. Glezen, W. P., W. A. Clyde, Jr., R. J. Senior et

al. 1967. Group A streptococci, mycoplasmas, and viruses associated with acute pharyngitis. *JAMA* 202:455–60.

7. Honikman, L. H., and B. F. Massell. 1971. Guidelines for the selective use of throat cultures in the diagnosis of streptococcal respiratory infection. *Pediatrics* 48:573–82.

8. Kaplan, E. L., F. H. Top, Jr., B. A. Dudding et al. 1971. Diagnosis of streptococcal pharyngitis: Differentiation of active infection from the carrier state in the symptomatic child. *J Infect Dis* 123:490–501.

9. Ross, P. W. 1971. Accuracy of clinical assessment of the microbial etiology of sore throat. *Practitioner* 207:659–61.

10. Rowe, R. T., and R. T. Stone. 1977. Streptococcal pharyngitis in children. Difficulties in diagnosis on clinical grounds alone. *Clin Pediatr* 16:933–35.

11. Commission on Acute Respiratory Diseases. 1944. Endemic exudative pharyngitis and tonsillitis. Etiology and clinical characteristics. *JAMA* 125:1163–69.

12. Brink, W. R., C. H. Rammelkamp, F. W. Denny et al. 1951. Effect of penicillin and aureomycin on the natural course of streptococcal tonsillitis and pharyngitis. *Am J Med* 10:300–08.

13. Wannamaker, L. W., C. H. Rammelkamp, Jr., F. W. Denny et al. 1951. Prophylaxis of acute rheumatic fever by treatment of the preceding streptococcal infection with various amounts of depot penicillin. *Am J Med* 10:673–95.

14. Walsh, B. T., W. W. Bookheim, R. C. Johnson et al. 1975. Recognition of streptococcal pharyngitis in adults. *Arch Intern Med* 135:1493–97.

15. Stillerman, M., and S. H. Bernstein. 1961. Streptococcal pharyngitis. Evaluation of clinical syndromes in diagnosis. *Am J Dis Child* 101:476–89.

16. Matanoski, G. M., W. H. Price, and C. Ferencz. 1968. Epidemiology of streptococcal infections in rheumatic and nonrheumatic families. II. The interrelationship of streptococcal infections to age, family transmission and type of group A. *Am J Epidemiol* 87:190–206.

17. Forsyth, R. S. 1975. Selective utilization of clinical diagnosis in treatment of pharyngitis. *J Fam Pract* 2:173–77.

18. El Kholy, A., D. W. Fraser, N. Guirguis et al. 1980. A controlled study of penicillin therapy of group A streptococcal acquisitions in Egyptian families. *J Infect Dis* 141:759–71.

19. Amren, D. P. 1972. Unusual forms of streptococcal disease. In *Streptococci and Streptococcal Diseases*, 545–56. L. W. Wannamaker, and J. M. Matsen ed. New

York: Academic Press.

20. Breese, B. B., and C. B. Hall. 1978. *Beta Hemolytic Streptococcal Diseases*. Boston: Houghton Mifflin.

21. Powers, G. F., and P. L. Boisvert. 1944. Age as a factor in streptococcosis. *J Pediat* 25:481–504.

22. Alpert, J. J., M. R. Pickering, and R. J. Warren. 1966. Failure to isolate streptococci from children under the age of 3 years with exudative tonsillitis. *Pediatrics* 38:663–66.

# 5

# Epidemiology of Rheumatic Fever

## Discussion

DR. SHULMAN: I would like to solicit additional data that may support the finding of a declining incidence of rheumatic fever.

DR. SCHWARTZ: Twenty-three children with acute rheumatic fever were admitted to our local community hospital in Fairfax County, Virginia, over a ten-year period. All were white, middle-class children, all but one American-born. Fairfax County, Virginia, had a population in 1970 of 455,000 and 597,000 in 1980. Thirty percent of the population during this time was from five to 19 years old. In 1980 the median family income for residents of Fairfax County was $39,500, and in the same year there were 15.6 deaths per 100,000 adult residents caused by rheumatic heart disease.

Our data in middle-class white children strongly support the data from Baltimore and from Memphis. In 1970 we had eight children admitted with the diagnosis of acute rheumatic fever fulfilling the Jones Criteria. By the late 1970s, the disease was extraordinarily rare.

Of our children, 43% had migratory polyarthritis, 26% had carditis without polyarthritis, and another 26% had polyarthritis with carditis. One child (4%) had pure Sydenham's chorea. There were no cases of erythema marginatum or subcutaneous nodules. Two children had an antecedent scarlatiniform rash and five had a throat culture positive for group A strep. Of interest is that in this series, only two children had a sore throat severe enough to bring them to a doctor. In one of them, rheumatic fever appeared to develop despite oral therapy.

In summary, rheumatic fever is now very infrequent in middle-class white children in Fairfax County, Virginia.

DR. KOMAROFF: We performed some indirect calculations from the National Center for Health Statistics data in the late 1970s. Our interest was in estimating the attack rate of primary acute rheumatic fever in adult patients who sought care for pharyngitis. This is a different denominator than we have been talking about until now. The estimates we made in the late 1970s were an attack rate of roughly 1/10,000 untreated adult patients and 1/100,000 treated adult patients, not comparable to the 3% attack rate in untreated young adults from Warren Air Force Base studies 30 years ago.

DR. HOUSER: We did surveys in Cleveland similar to Leon Gordis's in Baltimore in 1964–67. The rates in less-than 19-year olds were 30/100,000 in 1964–65, which were similar to what Dr. Robert Quinn found in Nashville at that time. In 1966–67, using the same methodology, the rate dropped to 17.5/100,000, coincident with installation of a mail-in throat culture program. The culture program was used most heavily in the inner city, and this is where this big drop occurred over a two-year period, similar to Leon's findings. Now, anecdotally, there are no more cases of rheumatic fever in Cleveland.

DR. SHULMAN: I can provide my antecdotal experience from Chicago. In the late 1960s, La Rabida was still a rheumatic fever hospital with large numbers of cases. Upon my return to Chicago after nine years, I found that rheumatic fever is very rare in our pediatric population. Our 265-bed Children's Hospital has seen two bona fide cases of acute rheumatic fever in the last three-and-a-half years.

DR. BISNO: Dr. Sophie Levinson from Chicago recently published in the *Journal of Chronic Disease* the data from the Chicago Rheumatic Fever Registry. The curves are dramatic; since 1962 the rate of decline has been spectacular, according to those studies.

DR. SHULMAN: Are there any other data on rheumatic fever incidence in the United States?

DR. COCHI: I want to report a study by the Rhode Island Health Department, similar in scope to the study by Alan Bisno, which has been submitted for publication. They looked at the incidence in Rhode Island from 1976 to 1980 and found an incidence rate of 0.2/100,000 overall population.

DR. SCHWARTZ: The attack rate in Fairfax County ranged from 3/100,000 in 1970 to 0.5/100,000 in 1980.

DR. DENNY: Are these age-corrected figures?

DR. SCHWARTZ: They are expressed for children five to 19 and include only first attacks.

DR. SHULMAN: The figure 0.5/100,000 certainly has been mentioned on several occasions this morning.

DR. STOLLERMAN: In confirmation of Milton Markowitz's comments about the Third World at the recent Congress of Cardiology in Capetown, South Africa, the incidence rates of rheumatic fever in the Soweto suburb of Johannesburg were estimated to be 200–400 cases/100,000 per year. There were very similar estimates for Durban. Although validation of that base population is difficult, the investigators doing the studies were very knowledgeable and made a very good effort to use populations with community medicine programs that gave some confidence to the estimates.

DR. DENNY: I would like to ask those who are quoting such high rates for the Third World whether those rates are changing. For instance, in Cairo, it's my understanding that, while the rates are still very high, they are declining fairly rapidly. Lew, is that correct?

DR. WANNAMAKER: Well, that's the impression, but I don't think there are any rates I would hang my hat on.

DR. DENNY: What about the rest of the Third World?

DR. STOLLERMAN: In South Africa there is about a hundred-year lag in the rate at which the native agrarian population is being industrialized and housed in and around the major cities, so that if anything we might be seeing less good housing or greater concentrations of populations under crowded conditions.

DR. HOUSER: What happened in Israel in the late 1960s was very dramatic, with rates going down almost year by year.

DR. SANFORD: It's interesting that in Panama City, Panama, rheumatic fever in the more affluent populations has virtually disappeared as we have heard here. On the other hand, in the portion that really still live in very crowded slums, rheumatic fever still has really quite a high prevalence. One can't come up with numbers, but all of the cases of rheumatic fever come from very specific localized areas within Panama City.

DR. MORTIMER: In the northern district of Santiago, Chile, which has a population of about half a million (all age groups), rheumatic fever cases have gone from about 50 per year down to about five, according to the Director of Maternal and Child Health. They don't see much anymore.

DR. SHULMAN: It appears that we are beginning to

develop a picture that, even in the Third World countries where the incidence is high, there is a suggestion of declining rates in most of these areas.

DR. DENNY: Are any studies being done to methodically examine children, let's say five, ten, and 15 years of age, to assess the presence of rheumatic heart disease? It's conceivable that we don't have any clinical acute rheumatic fever but still have rheumatic fever that leads to heart disease. I'm not aware of any studies like this having been done in the last 23 years. I want to know if there is a comparable decline in rheumatic carditis resulting in rheumatic heart disease.

DR. SANFORD: In Panama, classic rheumatic mitral stenosis is not seen in private practice in the affluent population of Panama City but is still a very prevalent problem in the indigent.

DR. DENNY: That's strange, because mitral stenosis should still be seen in 50- and 60-year-old people in the United States.

DR. SANFORD: We don't see much classical mitral stenosis in 50- and 60-year-old people in the United States anymore.

DR. STOLLERMAN: It's becoming a geriatric disease. When we want to see mitral stenosis, we look at the population over 60; 50-year-olds surprisingly less commonly than we used to see; and 40-year-olds hardly at all.

DR. SHULMAN: Does anybody have any data on changes in incidence of juvenile mitral stenosis in Third World countries?

DR. STOLLERMAN: The number of valve replacements in Capetown and in Johannesburg in juveniles is still tremendous. They have so many that they really can't schedule them for valve replacements. If anything, the cardiologists there think the incidence might even be increased.

DR. KAPLAN: There is some very soft evidence from the World Health Organization that there are several developing countries in the socialist bloc, particularly Mongolia and North Korea, in which rheumatic fever is also falling quite remarkably.

DR. EICKOFF: I want to ask the discussants who were quoting the continuing high rates in Third World countries what, if any, preventative programs are in effect in those countries. Do patients receive medical care, are they treated with penicillin, is there any kind of primary prevention program, for example?

DR. KAPLAN: It depends very much on the country that you are talking about. Most efforts in those countries are really impeded by social, economic, and political considerations rather than medical needs. There are some very good programs in a number of countries around the world. There are some that are absolutely abysmal.

DR. EICKOFF: What happened in Israel?

DR. HOUSER: In Israel changes were coincident with Mike Davies instituting prophylaxis programs in the schools. On Cyprus, where there was a lot of rheumatic heart disease and rheumatic fever, a program was instituted in the schools and they saw again a dramatic decline. In this school program, nurses identified sore throats in the schools, and they were treated.

The other problem, which is a recurrent one, is that in Cyprus the standard of living went up tremendously once they got the wars decided between the Turks and the Greeks, coincident with the culture program. There was a decline associated with the program, but other things were happening at the same time.

DR. MORTIMER: In the Cuyahoga County coroner's office, where enormous numbers of careful autopsies are done, rheumatic heart disease as a primary cause of death is just not seen anymore.

DR. DURACK: We have figures mainly on incidence and death rates. Does anybody in the audience have figures, not impressions, on the prevalence of valvular rheumatic disease in the United States? Is any such study underway or does anyone have the answer on prevalence?

DR. MARKOWITZ: A number of surveys of school children were done back in the 1960s in Chicago. Even in the early 1960s the prevalence of rheumatic heart disease among school children in the United States was really quite low. I don't think anybody has repeated that because it doesn't seem to be cost-effective to do those kinds of screening studies anymore.

DR. STOLLERMAN: Bob Miller's figure was about 1/1000 in the survey done in the 1960s among school children in Chicago. At that time the prevalence of rheumatic heart disease had just fallen below that of congenital heart disease.

DR. BISNO: I want to ask whether anyone has any data on the incidence of strep throat. If the incidence of rheumatic fever is falling, does that mean that the incidence of strep throat is falling, or does it mean that there are some changes in the host or the organism that relate to this decline? Leon Gordis speculated that the incidence of strep throat may be declining, too, to explain this. I have no hard data on this, but my general impression from the percentage of group A strep cultured from children with sore throats and from mean ASO population data is that there really is no evidence that strep throat is declining at all. Does anyone around the table have data or comments on that?

DR. SCHWARTZ: There is no difference in the incidence of strep throat over my 13 years of white middle-class pediatric practice. In Rochester, New York, where there are carefully obtained data, there is no difference.

DR. STOLLERMAN: In a recent small study of young adults at the Boston University Hospital Emergency Room, 10% of the people who came in with pharyngitis through the year had a positive culture.

DR. DILLON: Culture data from children in Birmingham, Alabama, who have had acute pharyngitis cultured using essentially the same criteria over the past 18 years indicate that the recovery of group A streptococcus is within 1%–2% over this period of time.

DR. HILL: Is there any change in the percentage of M-typeability or any other evidence of change in the streptococcus?

DR. MARKOWITZ: Dr. Quinn's earlier surveys over long-time periods showed a decline in M-typeability. Many of those cultured were healthy school children.

DR. DILLON: I can comment on the typing experience. We have not done extensive typing each year over the past 18 years. But there has been a fairly consistent 40%–43% M-typeability of strains recovered from children with acute pharyngitis entered into clinical studies over the years. Several years ago I presented some data at the Lancefield Society meeting in which we had compared our prevalent M-types in pharyngeal infection with those from Breese and Disney's group. Their M-typeability was 4%–5% greater than ours, but the prevalent types were not dissimilar.

In this respect, I think the data from Rochester are the best available regarding year-to-year changes in incidence of positive cultures and also scarlet fever incidence over the last 10–15 years. About three or four years ago, they noted an increase in scarlet fever in Rochester; this was associated with an increase in Type 3. About a year or two after that, we experienced an increase in scarlet fever, and we also saw a sharp increase in Type 3. That was the first time that we have had very many Type 3 infections. So there are changes in the prevalence of types, but overall percent typeability hasn't changed much.

DR. SHULMAN: Dr. Facklam, do you have data to add?

DR. FACKLAM: M-typeability for throat culture strains that were submitted to the Centers for Disease Control in potential epidemics has not changed in the past 16 years, remaining right at 40%.

DR. STOLLERMAN: I have looked at plates of group A streptococci for many years, including at the peak of epidemics in military populations. In the past 18 months that I have been looking at strep again, I have not seen anything like a big encapsulated mucoid strain in the population. I for one do not believe that M-typeability alone is a reflection of the nature of those strain variants. I wonder if anybody else still sees great big colonies.

DR. DILLON: The Type 3s that we are seeing resemble the classical old mucoid colonies that I saw in the J.E.M. pictures 30 years ago.

DR. SCHWARTZ: I read plates almost daily, and I agree that the mucoid type of strep colonies are very, very rare now. Even though we see a lot of beta-hemolytic strep, the typical mucoid colonies are not as common as they were eight or ten years ago.

DR. DENNY: I would like to ask Leon Gordis a question because the incidence of strep infection is not changing and obviously a change in the relationship between the strep-tococcus and the host is occurring. You discarded out of hand the possibility that the host was changing?

DR. SHULMAN: I believe that Dr. Gordis discounted significant genetic change during that period, rather than all host factors.

DR. DENNY: If you are talking about genetic factors, of course, I would agree with that. But it seems to me, with the decline of rheumatic fever beginning a fair period of time before the advent of either sulfonamides or penicillin, that there could have been a great deal of change in the hosts.

DR. MARKOWITZ: I wonder if some of you, as I, have been struck by the rapid change over the last 15 years? I think you can take this 30-year period and divide it into two 15-year periods. From 1950 to about 1965, there was still a fair amount of rheumatic fever. In the last 15 years, there has really been a striking acceleration. You have to look at what might have happened in the last 15 years. I would like to think that what has happened in the last 15 years is food stamps, Medicaid accessibility, availability of health care for kids. Poor children now get to the health care facility much more frequently than in the past. Maybe they are getting only three days of treatment or five days of treatment or whatever. But I can't escape the fact that there has been a marked decline in rheumatic fever in the last 15 years. We are down to a tiny, tiny number, and that's quite different from the curve that started in 1900. We don't know the role of nutrition relative to strep infections, but I suspect that this may be playing a role. These are environmental changes, which affect the host.

DR. TARANTA: It almost seems to me that the equilibrium is an unstable one between the streptococcus and the host. Therefore, a slight increase in medical care would not cause only a slight decrease in rheumatic fever. No, there is an equilibrium point at the left of which a kind of catastrophe occurs, a catastrophe of streptococcus. Nothing has happened in the last ten years that we can see, either in medical care or in socioeconomic changes, that parallels a tenfold decrease. I think we should use a different model, a catastrophe model in which the equilibrium was stable but now is catastrophic.

DR. BISNO: I think that too little has been made of changes in the organism in the past. I was not around in the era of the big mucoid streptococci, but there are data from a number of sources now indicating that all strep are not equal in terms of their ability to produce rheumatic fever. The evidence that Type 5 has something special about its ability to produce rheumatic fever is absolutely unequivocal. In southeast Santiago, Chile, we see 30 to 50 cases of rheumatic fever per year. I find Type 5 antibody in one-third of the kids with acute rheumatic fever, and we culture Type 5 from a lot of them. A very important factor in the equation must be related to the strain. The data are almost unassailable now that at least there are certain types that are very highly rheumatogenic and certain types that are very poorly rheumatogenic. For the great majority of types, one cannot say at this time. This raises the question that if indeed we could find the critical variable that relates to rheumatogenicity, whether it be the type or whatever, we might in the future be able to do something much more selective to prevent rheumatic fever than going out to hunt for every streptococcus in the world when it's clear that the risks are so low in many places now.

DR. AYOUB: How can you reconcile this with your observations and those of Leon Gordis regarding the high frequency of rheumatic fever in certain populations? Does that mean that Type 5 plays a major role in certain populations or environments?

DR. BISNO: I really can't say. We know that streptococci are much more virulent in environments that facilitate rapid person-to-person transmission. We have wondered for many years whether there might be microepidemics of virulent strains of group A streptococci causing some of these cases in the inner city. We have never really been able to demonstrate that here. So we have had to go to places like Chile, where there is a lot more rheumatic fever, to try to get some answers.

DR. HOUSER: I would like to comment on the risk of rheumatic fever following subclinical streptococcal infections. These are not hard data, but as we all get older, hardness becomes relative. In a study at Sampson Air Force Base, we knew the subclinical infection rate because we followed airmen longitudinally and identified an infection by isolation of group A strep and antibody response. We knew whether they had symptoms because they were evaluated, so we had a handle on the subclinical infection rate. We then looked at rheumatic fever and identified those rheumatics who had no evidence of clinical infection. The proportion of rheumatics who had had subclinical or asymptomatic streptococcal infections was the same as the proportion of subclinical infections present on the base during that same interval. This is the only information I am aware of that relates subclinical infections to the risk of rheumatic fever. The risks seem to be equal for subclinical and for symptomatic infections.

DR. MORTIMER: A question for Dr. Wannamaker: In terms of selectivity of whom you culture and whom you don't, under conditions of epidemic streptococcal disease or explosive outbreak, such as at the Air Force Academy, are the individuals who get streptococcal pharyngitis more apt to display the so-called classic features? As I look at the four or five studies reported in the old literature (and there isn't much endemic and epidemic streptococcal disease untreated with penicillin), the rates of rheumatic fever found with endemic disease are one-fifth to one-tenth those of epidemic streptococcal disease. I think that this difference is unlikely to be explained by dilution with carriers.

DR. WANNAMAKER: Well, I think that's one factor, but it may not be the only one. Certainly, in the food-borne epidemic at the Air Force Academy, the young men who were sick were really sick, with a lot of toxicity.

One fact that has been brought up before is that there was no rheumatic fever in these young men, but they were all treated with penicillin. Whether that is the explanation or not, we don't know. I think there were some cases of rheumatic fever in children either just before or just after that period, providing at last some indirect suggestion that the strain was rheumatogenic.

I don't think we really have the information to answer your question, Ted.

DR. DENNY: I'm concerned about the discussion of the clinical diagnosis of streptococcal infection and the fact that the data are being collected from patients presenting for medical care. Are we ever going to learn anything about the diagnosis of streptococcal infections until we do prospective population studies? Don't we need to culture every person of every age in that population, whether or not they have any respiratory disease, and follow them along? If we look only at who comes to the pediatrician's office, the study is biased before it gets started.

DR. WANNAMAKER: There are exceptions, of course, as the military population studies. In our study at Warren Air Force Base, we followed young men prospectively with cultures every day for long periods, sometimes several months. One can get some information from such studies. Transitory carriers were extremely common, particularly in the nose.

We also saw apparently subclinical infections. About two-thirds of the men had acquired a new type of group A strep and did not exhibit any symptomatology (at least that they would admit to) of streptococcal pharyngitis. One of the surprising things was that we saw tonsillitis in some young men who denied symptoms.

DR. DENNY: How many of these asymptomatic patients developed an antibody response?

DR. WANNAMAKER: There were fewer than those who had symptoms, you know, but these were not large groups, so the figures are not as reliable as one would like.

DR. HOUSER: In our studies at Sampson, 18% of the total streptococcal infections, defined as isolation of group A and an antibody response, were what we called asymptomatic or subclinical. We were looking for symptoms every other day.

DR. AYOUB: I like Dr. Denny's proposal about prospective studies. The only thing that's always asked whenever this is proposed is what to do with those who are found to be positive. Should they be treated or not and how would that influence your observations?

DR. DENNY: I hope this conference comes to grips with that question, because if we don't have to treat any streptococcal infection, God knows we don't have to treat asymptomatic ones.

DR. GERBER: Over the last several years in Connecticut, I have been impressed both with how infrequently I have seen scarlet fever and with how frequently that diagnosis is made by young physicians in patients who clearly don't have scarlet fever. I'm wondering if perhaps young physicians are no longer able to make the diagnosis of scarlet fever reliably because they no longer see this disease.

## STREPTOCOCCAL PHARYNGITIS IN INFANTS

DR. GERBER: Dr. Wannamaker, you alluded to work by Alpert and others demonstrating that the incidence of streptococcal pharyngitis in children younger than three years of age is quite low. I believe most of that work was done 20 or 25 years ago. With the dramatic increase in children attending day-care centers and nursery schools, has there been a change in the age-related incidence of streptococcal pharyngitis?

DR. WANNAMAKER: As far as I know there are no such data available. But perhaps others may have data on that point.

DR. DENNY: We have been following a day-care center population for a long time, and a diagnosis of streptococcal pharyngitis in a child under two is a rather unusual circumstance.

DR. WANNAMAKER: What about "streptococcal fever"?

DR. DENNY: I am getting on much more precarious ground now, because we haven't finished looking at our data. It would appear that the association between the acquisition of a group A streptococcus and symptomatology is a very weak one in children under two years of age and a very strong one over two years of age.

DR. WANNAMAKER: Well, that's exactly what Breese showed, but that doesn't mean the younger children didn't have a strep infection.

DR. DENNY: Absolutely. This does not mean that they did not have a serological response and a streptococcal infection.

DR. SHULMAN: Is "streptococcal fever" continuing to occur in its past described form?

DR. SCHWARTZ: I would like to comment on the incidence of positive cultures in the child under three. In the *Southern Medical Journal* a couple of years ago, we reported that 15% of young white middle-class children presenting with an acute URI, predominantly with red throat, had 2+ or greater positive throat cultures.

I see about one to two cases per year of acute streptococcosis or subacute streptococcal nasal pharyngitis.

DR. WANNAMAKER: I think one of the things we don't know is how common acute streptococcosis was when Powers and Boisvert were describing it. One gains the impression that it may have been common then, but there are no real data.

DR. McCARTY: I can comment on that point because it was something that in my pediatric day was discussed frequently at the Harriet Lane Home, but it wasn't seen there. I don't recall ever seeing a case of streptococcosis as described during my three years at Harriet Lane. I don't think it was common even then.

DR. BEEM: Do suppurative complications associated with group A strep in that age group provide an indirect index?

DR. WANNAMAKER: I can recall only one node that we drained in the past year that had a group A strep.

DR. DAJANI: My published data are quite old, but I think there has been a definite change in the etiology of acute cervical adenitis in that group A streptococci are now second to *Staphylococcus aureus*. When we looked at this in the early 1960s, there was a definite preponderance of group A streptococci.

DR. BEEM: I think some implications are starting to emerge regarding strep infections in very young children. What kind of illnesses are we sampling in this age group for strep? Are these children with any respiratory infection? We don't really get very reliable complaints of sore throat in children under two years of age. What is it that we are sampling for strep, and what are we going to do about it when we find it?

DR. MARKOWITZ: Dr. Schwartz, you had a 15% rate of culture positivity for group A beta-strep in children under age three, as I recall.

DR. SCHWARTZ: Yes. The reason the study got started was that, of four pediatricians in our group, two believed that children under age three could have positive throat cultures and did them routinely. Two, including myself, thought that the literature suggested it's not common. In fact, looking back at our data, it was 15% positive cultures for young children. Reviewing Breese's data, however, I was astounded to see that children between ten and 12 years of age had exactly 15% positive throat cultures, the same rate as that of children under three with exudative tonsillitis.

Our children were all symptomatic with upper respiratory infections, sometimes stuffy nose. On examination, the throat was red. Very few had a true exudate. On throat culture, only 2+ strep or greater was considered positive. Unfortunately, we have no serologic data. Most of the children seemed to improve with penicillin.

DR. WANNAMAKER: How do you exclude carriers?

DR. SCHWARTZ: I didn't. It could very well be they were all carriers.

DR. HILL: There is very little rheumatic fever in that age group, but there is a lot of nephritis. Doesn't some of that come from respiratory infection?

DR. DILLON: As a matter of fact, in children under five or six with nephritis, it's predominantly post-skin infection. In our experience, the mean age of nephritis following skin infection (five years) was about three years less than that following respiratory disease (eight years). The reported incidence of nephritis has been declining steadily. At Dr. Rammelkamp's commemorative meeting in Cleveland a few years ago, I presented our data from over about a 15-year period, beginning in the early 1960s, showing a sharp drop after about 8–10 years in the occurrence of nephritis. It's continued downward since then.

We also know that the three major nephritogenic streptococcal types we saw in those years are, for practical purposes, gone from our community.

DR. AMREN: Dr. Wannamaker, would it be safe to advise clinicians not to culture pharyngitis in children under two or three years of age? This would produce a tremendous cost savings if pediatricians and family practitioners accepted that there is very little or no risk of rheumatic fever in this group.

DR. WANNAMAKER: Well, it may be cost effective, but I guess I would hate to see that happen because it seems to me we need more information in this age group about how frequent strep infections are. If indeed there is something about an infection early in life that might relate to subsequent susceptibility to rheumatic fever, that might be entirely the wrong thing to do.

DR. AYOUB: I wonder whether Dr. Amren's suggestion applies especially to this country. Isn't the rate in developing countries higher in the younger age group? If we make statements like this, would they not then be hazardous to that population?

DR. SANFORD: I don't think the developing countries have cultured. I suspect it's very rare for a culture to be obtained under those circumstances.

# 6

# Diagnosis of Pharyngitis: Methodology of Throat Culture

*Michael A. Gerber, M.D.*

The signs and symptoms of group A beta-hemolytic strepto-coccal (GABHS) pharyngitis are nonspecific, making the clinical diagnosis of this disease, even for the most ex-perienced physician, unacceptably inaccurate. The per-formance of a throat culture is therefore essential for an accurate diagnosis. As most physicians are familiar with the procedure for performing a throat culture, no attempt will be made to review the specific details of the meth-odology. This discussion will instead concentrate on some of the more controversial aspects of the throat culture procedure.

DUPLICATE THROAT CULTURES

Despite the general acceptance of the throat culture as a diagnostic procedure, its reliability in identifying patients with GABHS in their upper respiratory tract has frequently been questioned. Several investigators have examined this issue by comparing duplicate throat cultures obtained at the time of the initial visit (Table 6–1). In 1954, Breese and Disney [1] performed duplicate throat cultures on patients with pharyngitis and found that the duplicate cultures were discordant in seven (8%) of the 85 patients, with at least one throat culture positive for GABHS. A single throat culture would therefore have missed 4% of the patients with GABHS in their upper respiratory tract. Stillerman and

TABLE 6-1. Concordance of Duplicate Throat Cultures

| Author | No. patients with pharyngitis and at least one of duplicate throat cultures positive | Percent of discordant throat cultures | Percent of positive patients missed with a single culture |
|---|---|---|---|
| Breese and Disney (1954) [1] | 85 | 8.0 | 4.0 |
| Stillerman and Bernstein (1961) [2] | 90 | 2.2 | 1.0 |
| Halfon et al. (1968) [3] | 343 | 24.0 | 12.0 |
| Kaplan et al. (1971) [4] | 133 | 0.0 | 9.0 |
| Kaplan et al. (1979) [5] | 50 | 12.0 | 6.0 |

Bernstein [2] performed a similar investigation and found that the duplicate throat cultures were discordant in only two (2.2%) of 90 pharyngitis patients with at least one throat culture positive for GABHS. Using a somewhat different approach, Moffet et al. [3] demonstrated a significant rise in ASO titer in only 11 of 306 patients (3.6%) with negative throat cultures and no antibiotic therapy, suggesting that few bona fide GABHS infections (defined as positive throat culture and serologic response to the GABHS) had been missed by a single throat culture.

In 1968, Halfon and co-workers [4] performed a series of throat cultures using two swabs simultaneously and then cultured each of the swabs separately on blood agar plates. They noted that in the 343 patients with at least one of the duplicate throat cultures positive for GABHS, a single culture would have missed approximately 12% of the positive patients. Kaplan et al. [5] performed duplicate throat cultures as part of their comprehensive study of acute pharyngitis in children in Minnesota. Despite vigorous swabbing of the pharynx and tonsils (or tonsillar fossae), they observed that 11 of the 133 children (9%) with at least one GABHS-positive throat culture would have been missed if only a single culture had been performed. Nine of these 11 patients had ten or fewer colonies of GABHS on their single positive culture, and the other two had fewer than 50 colonies. These data suggest that culture-positive patients who would have been missed on a single throat culture had fewer colonies of GABHS on the duplicate culture plate than patients whose duplicate cultures were both positive.

Recently, Kaplan and co-workers [6] reexamined this issue and found that six (12%) pairs of duplicate throat cultures were discordant in 50 patients with acute pharyngitis and at least one GABHS-positive throat culture. Therefore, a single throat culture would have missed three (6%) of the symptomatic, culture-positive patients. As in their earlier study, they found that the positive culture in the discordant pairs often had fewer than ten colonies of GABHS. Although the number of patients was small, the investigators were troubled by the facts that half of the patients with discordant throat cultures demonstrated a serologic response to the streptococci in their throats and that three of the 21 patients (14%) who demonstrated a serologic response and had had duplicate cultures performed had discordant duplicate throat cultures.

The discordance of duplicate cultures has been offered as evidence that the throat culture is unreliable as a diagnostic test. Review of existing data suggests, however, that although the discordance rate may be as high as 20%, only about one patient in ten with GABHS in the upper respiratory tract would be missed if a single throat culture were performed. Furthermore, these discordance rates are calculated on the basis of positive cultures only. Since one may expect at least two to three negative throat cultures for each positive one, the discordance rate for all throat cultures is actually 5% or less. In addition, for most of the discordant cultures, the positive culture was only weakly positive, suggesting that most of these patients may be carriers (positive throat culture without serologic response to the GABHS) and not truly infected (positive throat culture with serologic response to the GABHS).

## QUANTITATION OF THROAT CULTURES

Another controversial issue has been the significance of the quantitation of GABHS isolated from a throat culture. In 1958, Miller et al. [7] reported a definite relationship between the number of colonies of streptococci isolated from a throat culture and the frequency with which the patient from whom the throat culture was obtained demonstrated a significant increase in ASO titer. However, 55% of those with the heaviest growth of streptococci on throat culture did not demonstrate an ASO response. Several years later, Stillerman and Bernstein [2] found that throat cultures with 1+ to 2+ positivity for GABHS were much more common in asymptomatic children than in children with acute pharyngitis, while cultures with 4+ positivity were much more common in the symptomatic group. Cultures with 3+ positivity were seen with approximately equal frequency in both groups. In 1970, Breese et al. [8] noted a strong relationship between the degree of positivity of throat cultures and "significant clinical illness." They suggested that the more acute, characteristic, or severe the nature of the streptococcal pharyngitis, the higher the degree of positivity of the throat culture and that cultures with a low degree of positivity were usually "unimportant."

Kaplan and co-workers [5], in a study of 218 children with acute streptococcal pharyngitis, could not demonstrate a consistent relationship between the degree of positivity of the initial throat culture and the subsequent change in either the ASO or anti-DNAse B titer. In addition, they noted that approximately one-third of patients with fewer than ten colonies of GABHS on initial throat culture subsequently demonstrated a significant serologic response. In a study comparing throat culture results from 1,054 children with acute pharyngitis and 462 healthy children, Bell and Smith [9] isolated GABHS from 35% of those with pharyngitis and from 17% of healthy controls. In the group with pharyngitis, 71% of positive cultures contained a heavy growth of GABHS, while in healthy children only 10% of positive cultures showed a heavy growth. They also found that the clinical diagnosis of streptococcal pharyngitis had been accurately made in 81% of patients with heavy growth of GABHS on throat culture but in only 59% of patients with light growth.

In a reexamination of their earlier work, Kaplan et al. [6] studied quantitative throat cultures from 86 patients with acute pharyngitis and from 110 of their clinically normal family contacts. Three-plus cultures were obtained in 24 of 31 (77%) initial GABHS-positive symptomatic patients compared to only six of 22 (27%) initial GABHS-positive throat cultures from asymptomatic contacts. In addition, all 12 patients with a positive throat culture and a significant antibody rise in ASO and/or anti-DNAse B had an initial 3+ culture, while only 46% of the 41 patients with a positive throat culture but without a significant antibody rise had an initial 3+ culture.

These studies suggest that patients with pharyngitis are more likely to have strongly positive cultures than asymptomatic children; patients with severe pharyngitis are more likely to have strongly positive cultures than patients with mild pharyngitis; and patients with true streptococcal infections are more likely to have strongly positive cultures than streptococcal carriers. However, there is so much overlap that differentiation of patients with streptococcal infections from patients who are streptococcal carriers can not be accurately made on the basis of the degree of positivity of the throat culture alone.


ATMOSPHERE OF INCUBATION

There has also been a great deal of debate about which atmosphere of incubation—aerobic, 5% $CO_2$, or anaerobic—is best for the cultivation and identification of GABHS. In 1974, McGonagle [10] surveyed 304 throat cultures using three different incubation techniques: anaerobic, aerobic with an agar overlay, and aerobic surface streaking with subsurface stabs. She found that 22, 21, and 19 of GABHS and 33, 28, and 11 of the non-group A beta-hemolytic streptococci were isolated with the anaerobic, agar overlay, and streak/stab techniques, respectively. She also found that in 31 cultures in which GABHS were isolated after anaerobic incubation, almost half of the duplicate cultures incubated in 5% $CO_2$ had no beta-hemolytic organisms.

Murray and coworkers [11] inoculated approximately 300 throat cultures onto three separate blood agar plates with streaking and subsurface stabs. The three plates were then randomly incubated in either an aerobic, 3%–5% $CO_2$, or anaerobic atmosphere and the recovery rates of streptococci compared. Significantly more non-group A beta-hemolytic streptococci were isolated after anaerobic and 5% $CO_2$ incubation than after aerobic incubation. The recovery rates of GABHS, however, were not significantly different for the three atmospheres, after either 24 or 48 hours of incubation.

In a similar study, Dykstra et al. [12] streaked 1263 throat cultures onto two separate blood agar plates, which were then randomly incubated either anaerobically or aerobically with subsurface stabs. Of the 149 cultures with GABHS on at least one of the duplicate plates, 94 (63%) were positive after aerobic incubation and 146 (98%) were positive after anaerobic incubation. However, only 8% of the negative aerobic plates contained non-group A beta-hemolytic streptococci, while 31% of the negative anaerobic plates contained non-group A beta-hemolytic streptococci.

In 1979, Baron and Gates [13] performed throat cultures with duplicate swabs and then inoculated each swab onto a separate blood agar plate, one of which was incubated aerobically and the other in 5% $CO_2$. They found essentially no difference in the isolation rates of either group A or non-group A beta-hemolytic streptococci after incubation in either atmosphere. In a similar study, Pien et al. [14] inoculated 725 throat swabs onto two separate plates, one of which was incubated anaerobically and the other in 5% $CO_2$, with subsurface stabs. A significantly greater number of plates contained beta-hemolytic streptococci after anaerobic incubation. There was no significant difference, however, in the number of plates containing GABHS after incubation in either atmosphere. Interestingly, the plates incubated anaerobically required significantly more subculturing of suspicious colonies than did the plates incubated in 5% $CO_2$. Kurzynski and Van Holten [15] streaked 334 throat cultures with subsurface stabs onto two separate plates, which were then randomly incubated either anaerobically or in 5%–10% $CO_2$. GABHS were isolated from 91 and 78 of the anaerobic and $CO_2$ plates, respectively, and non-group A beta-hemolytic streptococci were isolated from 68 and 29 of the anaerobic and $CO_2$ plates, respectively. These studies are summarized in Table 6–2.

Anaerobic incubation of throat cultures is theoretically desirable for several reasons: inactivation of the oxygen-labile streptolysin O is prevented, peroxide production that can interfere with the expression of beta-hemolysis is inhibited, and the growth of aerobic normal throat flora is suppressed. It is therefore not surprising that several of the cited investigators [10,12,15] demonstrated a higher isolation rate of GABHS from throat cultures when anaerobic rather than 5% $CO_2$ or aerobic incubation is employed. However, as previously noted, other investigators [11,13, 14] have been unable to demonstrate a significant difference. Whether the increased number of patients with positive throat cultures, which could potentially result from anaerobic incubation, represents an increase in those with true streptococcal infections or merely an increased number of streptococcal carriers remains to be determined. It is also apparent that anaerobic incubation of throat cultures results in a higher isolation rate of non-group A beta-hemolytic streptococci and, in turn, a greater need for subculturing than either 5% $CO_2$ or aerobic incubation. The increased cost and effort of anaerobic incubation would

TABLE 6-2. Effect of Incubating Atmosphere on Isolation Rate of Beta-Hemolytic Streptococci

| Author | Group A | Non-Group A |
|---|---|---|
| McGonagle (1974) [10] | AN > AE <br> AN > $CO_2$ | AN > AE |
| Murray et al. (1976) [11] | AN = AE = $CO_2$ | AN > $CO_2$ > AE |
| Dykstra et al. (1979) [12] | AN > AE | AN > AE |
| Baron and Gates (1979) [13] | AE = $CO_2$ | AE = $CO_2$ |
| Pien et al. (1979) [14] | AN = $CO_2$ | AN = $CO_2$ |
| Kurzynski and Van Holten (1981) [15] | AN > $CO_2$ | AN > $CO_2$ |

AN = Anaerobic; AE = Aerobic; $CO_2$ = 5% $CO_2$

appear difficult to justify at this time, particularly for the physician processing throat cultures in his own office.

## BACITRACIN DIFFERENTIATION TEST

Probably the most widely used test for the identification of group A streptococci is the bacitracin differentiation test. This test provides a presumptive identification based on the observation that 95%–100% [16,17] of GABHS demonstrate a zone of inhibition around a disc containing 0.04 units of bacitracin, while 83%–97% of non-group A beta-hemolytic streptococci do not. Several recent attempts have been made to increase the accuracy of the bacitracin differentiation test.

Maxted [20], in his original description of the bacitracin disc test, made no mention of a minimal zone of inhibition in order for an organism to be considered bacitracin-sensitive. However, it has been suggested that requiring a 10 mm or greater zone of inhibition would increase the accuracy of the test. The package insert from one manufacturer of bacitracin discs still implies that zones of 10 mm or greater are necessary for the presumptive identification of GABHS.

In one of the few studies that addresses this question, Ederer et al. [17] examined 1197 strains of beta-hemolytic streptococci using 10 mm inhibition as the cutoff for bacitracin-sensitivity. She found that 561 (95.9%) of the 585 serologically confirmed GABHS were bacitracin-sensitive (false negative rate of 4.1%) and 87.3% of the non-group A beta-hemolytic streptococci were bacitracin-resistant (false positive rate of 12.7%). When any zone of inhibition was considered evidence of bacitracin-sensitivity, 100% of GABHS were bacitracin-sensitive. Murray and co-workers [16] observed that of 652 isolates of beta-hemolytic streptococci that demonstrated any zone of inhibition around a bacitracin disc, only 21 (3.2%) had inhibitory zones less than 10 mm.

In his original description, Maxted [20] also noted that if sufficient numbers of beta-hemolytic colonies were present, the bacitracin disc could be placed on the primary blood agar plate with accurate interpretation of results. Although most studies documenting the accuracy of the bacitracin disc test were performed on subcultures, placing the bacitracin disc on the primary blood agar plate has certain advantages: A one-day rather than a two-day delay in obtaining results, which increases patient satisfaction, elimination of the cost of subculturing, and better patient compliance. The only disadvantages are the cost of the disc (approximately $0.03/each), the additional few seconds it takes to drop the disc on the plate, and the potential for producing a false negative throat culture by inhibiting all the GABHS colonies on the primary plate. Over the years, there has been controversy regarding the accuracy and practicality of the bacitracin disc test when applied to primary blood agar plates. A review of three recent studies [16,21,22] shows that approximately 70% of cultures containing beta-hemolytic streptococci can be read properly after placement of the bacitracin disc on the primary blood agar plate and that only about 30% require subculturing (Table 6–3). In addition, with this method approximately half of the throat cultures with GABHS can be identified in 24 rather than 48 hours. However, one must consider primary plates with bacitracin discs unreadable if there are too few beta-hemolytic colonies in the area of the disc or if there are beta-hemolytic, bacitracin-resistant strains of normal oropharyngeal flora (for example, *Staphylococcus aureus*) obscuring the zone of inhibition of GABHS around the disc.

It has also been suggested that alteration of the incubating atmosphere might improve the accuracy of the bacitracin disc test. Maxted [20] observed that the dis-

TABLE 6-3. Identification of Group A Streptococci with Bacitracin Disc on Primary Throat Culture Plate

| Author | Cultures with Beta-Hemolytic Streptococci | Cultures with Group A | Cultures with Beta Strep Readable on Primary Plate | Cultures with Group A Readable on Primary Plate |
|---|---|---|---|---|
| Sprunt et al. (1974) [21] | 374 | -- | 264 (71%) | -- |
| Murray et al. (1976) [16] | 1,229 | 638 | 949 (77%) | 358 (56%) |
| Lyerly et al. (1980) [22] | 1,047 | 605 | 691 (65%) | 387 (64%) |

tinction between group A and non-group A streptococci was sharper under anaerobic conditions. However, in an atmosphere of increased $CO_2$ content, he found that the activity of bacitracin was increased equally against both group A and non-group A strains. Kurzynski and Van Holten [15] recently demonstrated that anaerobic incubation increased the number of GABHS that could be identified using the bacitracin disc test when compared to incubation in 5% $CO_2$. However, anaerobic incubation also increased the number of bacitracin-sensitive non-group A beta-hemolytic streptococci that were isolated and misidentified as group A. Beerman and Goldblatt [23] also recently showed that anaerobic incubation increased the number of GABHS that could be identified with a bacitracin disc on the primary blood agar plate when compared to aerobic incubation.

Others have attempted to increase the accuracy of the bacitracin differentiation test by combining the bacitracin disc with another antibiotic disc. For example, a disc containing 1.25 µg of trimethoprim and 23.75 µg of sulfamethoxazole (SXT) placed next to a bacitracin disc on the primary blood agar plate will inhibit the normal oropharyngeal flora in the area around the bacitracin disc and make it easier to visualize small numbers of GABHS. Kurzynski and Van Holten et al. [15] noted that the combination of bacitracin and SXT discs produced primary plates that were more often readable than when bacitracin discs were used alone. Since GABHS are usually bacitracin-sensitive and SXT-resistant, group B beta-hemolytic streptococci are usually bacitracin-resistant and SXT-resistant, and other non-group A beta-hemolytic streptococci are usually bacitracin-resistant and SXT-sensitive, the sensitivity patterns of a subculture of beta-hemolytic streptococci to both discs can be used to differentiate group A from non-group A streptococci. Gunn [24] found that the sensitivity and specificity of the bacitracin disc on a subculture of beta-hemolytic streptococci to be 100% and 88%, respectively, but increase to 99% and 99%, respectively, when used in conjunction with a SXT disc.

In summary, the measurement of the zone of inhibition around the bacitracin disc is not necessary for the differentiation of group A from non-group A beta-hemolytic streptococci. Zones less than 10 mm appear to occur infrequently, and the increased incidence of false positive cultures that might occur if zones are not measured is more than compensated for by the increased sensitivity of the test. If interpreted properly, the placement of the bacitracin disc on the primary blood agar plate can expedite and reduce the cost of the throat culture procedure. Anaerobic incubation may increase the sensitivity of the bacitracin differentiation test but, at the same time, may decrease the specificity of the test. More data are required to determine whether the additional effort and cost of anaerobic incubation can be justified in this situation. Finally, the use of other antibiotic discs in conjunction with the bacitracin disc to increase the accuracy of the differentiation test appears promising.

REFERENCES

1. Breese, B. B., and F. A. Disney. 1954. The accuracy of diagnosis of beta streptococcal infections on clinical grounds. *J Pediatr* 44:670.

2. Stillerman, M., and S. H. Bernstein. 1961. Streptococcal pharyngitis: Evaluation of clinical syndromes in diagnosis. *Am J Dis Child* 101:476.

3. Moffet, H. L., H. G. Cramblett, and J. P. Black. 1964. Group A streptococcal infections in a children's home: I. Evaluation of practical bacteriologic methods. *Pediatrics* 33:5.

4. Halfon, S. T., A. M. Davies, O. Kaplan et al. 1968. Primary prevention of rheumatic fever in Jerusalem school children: II. Identification of beta-hemolytic streptococci. *Isr J Med Sci* 4:809.

5. Kaplan, E. L., F. H. Top, Jr., B. A. Dudding et

al. 1971. Diagnosis of streptococcal pharyngitis: Differentiation of active infection from the carrier state in symptomatic children. *J Infect Dis* 123:490.

6. Kaplan, E. L., R. Couser, B. B. Huwe et al. 1979. Significance of quantitative salivary cultures for group A and non-group A beta-hemolytic streptococci in patients with pharyngitis and their family contacts. *Pediatrics* 64:904.

7. Miller, J. M., S. L. Stancer, and B. F. Massell. 1958. A controlled study of beta-hemolytic streptococcal infection in rheumatic families. I. Streptococcal disease among healthy siblings. *Am J Med* 25:825.

8. Breese, B. B., F. A. Disney, W. B. Talpey et al. 1970. Beta-hemolytic streptococcal infection. The clinical and epidemiologic importance of the number of organisms found in cultures. *Am J Dis Child* 119:18.

9. Bell, S. M., and D. D. Smith. 1976. Quantitative throat-swab culture in the diagnosis of streptococcal pharyngitis in children. *Lancet* 2:61.

10. McGonagle, L. A. 1974. Evaluation of a screening procedure for the isolation of beta-hemolytic streptococci. *Health Lab Sci* 11:61.

11. Murray, P. R., A. D. Wold, C. A. Schreck et al. 1976. Effects of selective media and atmosphere of incubation on the isolation of group A streptococci. *J Clin Microbiol* 4:54.

12. Dykstra, M. A., J. C. McLaughlin, and R. C. Bartlett. 1979. Comparison of media and techniques for detection of group A streptococci in throat swab specimens. *J Clin Microbiol* 9:236.

13. Baron, E. J., and J. W. Gates. 1979. Primary plate identification of group A beta-hemolytic streptococci utilizing a two-disk technique. *J Clin Microbiol* 10:80.

14. Pien, F. D., C. L. Ow, N. S. Isaacson et al. 1979. Evaluation of anaerobic incubation for recovery of group A streptococci from throat cultures. *J Clin Microbiol* 10:392.

15. Kurzynski, T. A., and C. M. Van Holten. 1981. Evaluation of techniques for isolation of group A streptococci from throat cultures. *J Clin Microbiol* 13:891.

16. Murray, P. R., A. D. Wold, M. M. Hall et al. 1976. Bacitracin differentiation for presumptive identification of group A beta-hemolytic streptococci: Comparison of primary and purified plate testing. *J Pediatr* 89:576.

17. Ederer, G. M., M. M. Herrmann, R. Bruce et al. 1972. Rapid extraction method with pronase B for grouping beta-hemolytic streptococci. *Appl Microbiol* 23:285.

18. Levinson, M. L., and P. F. Frank. 1955. Differentiation of group A from other beta-hemolytic streptococci

with bacitracin. *J Bacteriol* 69:284.

19. Facklam, R. R., J. F. Padula, and C. G. Thacker. 1974. Presumptive identification of group A, B, and D streptococci. *Appl Microbiol* 27:107.

20. Maxted, W. R. 1953. The use of bacitracin for identifying group A hemolytic streptococci. *J Clin Path* 6:224.

21. Sprunt, K., D. Vail, and R. S. Asnes. 1974. Identification of *Streptococcus pyogenes* in a pediatric outpatient department: A practical system designed for rapid results and resident teaching. *Pediatrics* 54:718.

22. Lyerly, W. H., J. W. Bass, and L. B. Harden. 1980. Identification of group A streptococci with bacitracin disc on the primary throat culture plate. *J Pediatr* 96:431.

23. Beerman, C. A., and S. A. Goldblatt. 1982. Screening for group A streptococcus by means of anaerobic primary plate technique. *J Pediatr* 101:70.

24. Gunn, B. A. 1976. SXT and Taxo A disks for presumptive identification of group A and B streptococci in throat cultures. *J Clin Microbiol* 4:192.

# 7

# Diagnosis and Treatment of Streptococcal Pharyngitis: Survey of U.S. Medical Practitioners

*Stephen L. Cochi, M.D., David W. Fraser, M.D., Allen W. Hightower, M.S., Richard R. Facklam, Ph.D., and Claire V. Broome, M.D.*

A recent controversy has developed between physicians who feel that all persons with a sore throat should have a throat culture to detect group A streptococci and those who feel that considerations of cost, sensitivity, and specificity of culturing make it better strategy to omit culturing in most instances of sore throat [1–8]. Traditionally, an important justification for widespread throat culturing has been the prevention of acute rheumatic fever (ARF), but this disease has now become rare in the United States [9–14]. Reassessment of the classical approach to the diagnosis and treatment of streptococcal pharyngitis therefore seems appropriate.

In addition to their role in primary prevention of ARF, throat cultures have been promoted to limit unnecessary use of antibiotics, to assist in defining and limiting transmission of group A streptococci and to provide data on the prevalence of this organism in the community. However, throat cultures are an imperfect tool because they identify asymptomatic carriers in addition to patients with active streptococcal disease, and these false positive cultures result in overtreatment. Taking a single throat culture has also been shown to have an 8%–12% false negative rate. Despite these limitations, the use of throat cultures to establish the diagnosis of streptococcal pharyngitis has been nationally recommended [15].

To limit overuse of throat cultures, guidelines based on clinical and epidemiologic features have been suggested for the selective use of throat cultures for diagnosis [15–24], and management strategies [17,25]. There is no recent published information available regarding the actual practices of U.S. primary care physicians; the only available information is restricted to pediatric and general practitioners in Baltimore [26], and to primary care physicians in Rhode Island [27]. An assessment of current practices is relevant to the evaluation of current resource utilization, particularly because sore throat is one of the most common problems seen in medical practice. Symptoms referable to the throat represent the third leading reason given by patients for office visits in the United States, amounting to nearly 27 million (4.7%) of over 577 million total visits per year [28]. Unnecessary culturing of these patients would result in substantial costs. Evidence has been presented that growth in the collective expenses of tests and procedures performed in managing common illnesses is a major contributing factor in escalating health costs [29].

Although the role of the throat culture in the management of streptococcal pharyngitis has been debated in the recent medical literature [1–8], the effect of this debate on physician practices in the United States is unknown. Our study was designed to assess current practices in a systematic fashion, using a mailed questionnaire survey of a random sample of U.S. medical practitioners.

METHODS

Study Population

The respondent universe consisted of all 107,201 nonfederal U.S. physicians whose primary specialty was family practice, general practice, internal medicine, or pediatrics, and whose major professional activity was in direct patient care or medical teaching (Table 7–1). Physicians still in residency training were excluded from the survey. The respondent universe was obtained from the AMA Physician Masterfile [30]. The survey sample was taken from file data for November 1982. A systematic stratified random sample of 500 physicians was obtained from each of three specialty groups: general and family practitioners (FP/GP), internists (IM), and pediatricians (PD).

Description of Survey

The 1500 medical practitioners identified by random sampling were mailed questionnaires in December 1982. Nonrespond-

TABLE 7-1. Distribution of U.S. Primary Care Physicians, November 1982, by Primary Specialty

| Primary specialty | Number of physicians |
|---|---|
| Family practice (FP) | 24,301 |
| General practice (GP) | 27,896 |
| Internal medicine (IM) | 36,481 |
| Pediatrics (PD) | 18,523 |
| Total respondent universe | 107,201 |

ents received a follow-up mailing one month later, consisting of the same questionnaire and a letter requesting cooperation. Data collection was completed three weeks after the second mailing.

The survey contained questions regarding demographic characteristics of the physician and his or her practice, procedures for the evaluation of patients with sore throat, methods for diagnosis, availability and cost of these methods, and therapy. Survey results were tabulated by specialty group, and a weighted average of the results was determined for the entire universe of primary care physicians from which the survey sample was drawn. Each weighted average was calculated in the same manner by weighting the response of an individual specialty group according to the proportion of the universe that specialty group comprised. Thus, the response of the group of family and general practitioners was weighted more heavily than that of internists or pediatricians in computing the weighted average. When using the weighted average results to define the practices of all primary care physicians, the practices of nonrespondents were assumed to be identical to those of respondent physicians. All percentages for each variable were derived from the number of respondents who answered and were rounded to the nearest whole number.

Survey of Private and Hospital Laboratories

A telephone survey of a nonrandom sample of ten private and ten hospital laboratories in metropolitan Atlanta was performed to determine laboratory throat culture methods and charges, for comparison with the physician survey results and to validate these results.


RESULTS

The overall response rate to the survey of primary care practitioners was 38% (570/1500) (Table 7–2). Three respondents did not fall into a primary care specialty group, and were excluded from the analysis. For the remaining 567 respondents, the response was greatest for pediatricians (45%), followed by family and general practitioners (35%), and internists (34%). A problem with this study was the relatively low response rate and the issue of whether respondents were a representative sample. However, board certification rates of respondents appeared to be representative of the study population. Pediatrician respondents were more likely to be board-certified (71%), than internist respondents (52%), or family and general practitioner respondents (41%) ($p < 0.001$). These rates of certification are similar to 1980 data on all non-federal U.S. physicians for these specialty groups: pediatrics (55%), internal medicine (49%), family and general practice (35%) [30]. Survey respondents were only slightly more likely to be board-certified than their peers for all three specialty groups. Also, the practice setting in which respondents saw the majority of their patients appeared to be representative, and was distributed as shown in Table 7–3. Physician respondents represented 46 states and the District of Columbia. The median age of respondents was 48 years, with a range from 26–83 years. Ninety-eight percent of respondents held the M.D. degree and 2% the D.O. degree. Graduates of foreign medical schools were overrepresented among respondents (Table 7–4), comprising approximately 41% of the weighted average response of primary care physicians although they constituted about 18% of the respondent universe in 1980 [30]. However, when survey results were stratified by foreign medical graduates versus U.S. graduates, no statistically significant differences in responses were observed.

Family and general practitioners reported that they saw an average of 116 patients per week in 1982, while pediatricians saw an average of 111 patients per week, and internists saw 74 patients per week (Table 7–5). The diagnosis of acute pharyngitis was made in approximately 24 patients per week by family and general practitioners, 23 per week by pediatricians, and 9 per week by internists

TABLE 7-2. Physician Survey Response Rate by Specialty Group and Board Certification

| Primary specialty | Percentage of respondents | | | Percentage total response |
| | Board certified | Not Board certified | Total (N) | |
| --- | --- | --- | --- | --- |
| Family practice/ general practice | 41 | 59 | 100 (175) | 35 |
| Internal medicine | 52 | 48 | 100 (168) | 34 |
| Pediatrics | 71* | 29 | 100 (224) | 45 |
| Totals | | | (567) | 38 |

*p < .001 ($\chi^2$=35.79,df=2)
Conservative 95% confidence limits: FP/GP±8%, IM±8%, PD±7%


TABLE 7-3. Primary Specialty of Physician Respondents by Practice Setting (percentage)

| Practice setting | Primary specialty | | | Weighted average all primary care |
| | FP/GP | IM | PD | |
| --- | --- | --- | --- | --- |
| Private office | 90 | 83 | 75 | 85 |
| Hospital based office/clinic | 5 | 7 | 16 | 7 |
| Health center | 1 | 2 | 2 | 1 |
| Emergency room | 1 | 2 | 0 | 1 |
| H.M.O. | 1 | 3 | 6 | 2 |
| Other | 3 | 2 | 1 | 3 |
| Totals | 100 | 100 | 100 | 100 |

Conservation 95% confidence limits: by specialty, FP/GP±8%, IM±8%, PD±7%, for weighted averages ±5%

TABLE 7-4.  Physician Survey Response Rate by Specialty Group and FMG vs U.S. Graduate Physicians

| Primary specialty | Percentage of Respondents | | |
| --- | --- | --- | --- |
| | FMG | U.S. grad | Total |
| Family practice/ general practice | 33* | 67 | 100 |
| Internal medicine | 49 | 51 | 100 |
| Pediatrics | 45 | 55 | 100 |
| Weighted average | 41 | 59 | 100 |

*p = .0063 ($\chi^2$=10.14,df=2)
Conservative 95% confidence limits: by specialty, FP/GP±8%, IM±8%, PD±7%, for weighted averages ±5%

TABLE 7-5.  Average Number of Patients Seen per Physician per Week (1982), by Primary Specialty

| Primary specialty | | Mean number of patients seen per physician per week | | |
| --- | --- | --- | --- | --- |
| | | (< 18 yr) Children | (≧ 18 yr) Adults | Total |
| Family practice/ general practice | (N = 167) | 34 (±5) | 83 (±7) | 116 (±9) |
| Internal medicine | (N = 160) | 5 (±2) | 69 (±5) | 75 (±6) |
| Pediatrics | (N = 213) | 106 (±7) | 5 (±2) | 111 (±7) |

Numbers in parentheses (±N) = ±2 Standard error

(Table 7–6). These figures are derived, in most cases, from individual estimates of respondent physicians rather than exact data from billing or survey records, and are intended to be estimates only.

The physician's specialty appeared to be a more important factor than the age of the patient in determining whether a patient with acute pharyngitis was cultured. Children (< 18 years of age) with acute pharyngitis who were seen by pediatricians were most likely to have a throat culture taken (66%), compared with internists (46%), or family and general practitioners (37%) (Table 7–7). Adults with acute pharyngitis who were seen by pediatricians were also more likely to have a throat culture taken (65%), compared with internists (34%), or family and general practitioners (28%). Pediatricians reported obtaining an average of 16 throat cultures per physician per week in 1982, while family and general practitioners obtained an average of six, and internists an average of three (Table 7–8).

Approximately 25% of primary care practitioners always or nearly always obtained throat cultures from their patients with acute sore throat, while 23% never or almost never obtained cultures (Table 7–9). Pediatricians were significantly more likely (54%) to always or nearly always obtain a throat culture from a patient with acute sore throat regardless of the patient's other symptoms, physical findings, demographic characteristics, or historic characteristics, when compared with internists (16%) or family and general practitioners (18%) ($p < 0.0001$). Correspondingly, pediatricians were least likely (5%) to never obtain a throat culture from such patients, when compared with internists (28%) or family and general practitioners (36%). Throat cultures were selectively obtained by 52% of primary care physicians. All specialty groups were similar in the proportion of respondents who selectively used throat cultures.

The 260 physicians who selectively obtained throat cultures were asked to rate the importance of individual symptoms, signs, demographic, and historic characteristics, from a list provided, in their assessment of the patient with acute sore throat. Three ratings were provided: (1) decisive = sufficient evidence by itself to convince the physician to obtain a throat culture, (2) suggestive = would only be sufficient evidence to obtain a throat culture in combination with one or more other items, and (3) not helpful = of no use to the physician in deciding whether to obtain a throat culture. The American Heart Association (AHA) [15] lists tender anterior cervical lymph nodes,

TABLE 7-6.  Average Number of Patients with Acute Pharyngitis Seen per Physician per Week (1982), by Primary Specialty

| Primary specialty | | Mean number of patients with acute pharyngitis seen per physician per week | | |
| --- | --- | --- | --- | --- |
| | | (< 18 yr) Children | (≧ 18 yr) Adults | Total |
| Family practice/ general practice | (N = 161) | 10 (±2) | 14 (±2) | 24 (±3) |
| Internal medicine | (N = 157) | 2 (±2) | 7 (±2) | 9 (±3) |
| Pediatrics | (N = 207) | 22 (±7) | 1 (±0.8) | 23 (±8) |

Numbers in parentheses (±N) = ±2 Standard error

TABLE 7-7.  Average Percentage of Acute Pharyngitis Patients from Whom a Throat Culture Was Obtained, by Primary Specialty and Age Group

| Primary specialty | Mean percentage of acute pharyngitis patients from whom a throat culture was obtained | |
| --- | --- | --- |
| | (< 18 yr) Children (N) | (≧ 18 yr) Adults (N) |
| Family practice/ general practice 95% C.I. | 37 (141) ±5.9 | 28 (137) ±5.4 |
| Internal medicine 95% C.I. | 46 (73) ±8.4 | 34 (147) ±5.1 |
| Pediatrics 95% C.I. | 66 (210) ±4.7 | 65 (62) ±9.4 |

95% C.I. = width of 95% confidence limits

TABLE 7-8. Average Number of Throat Cultures Obtained per Physician per Week (1982), by Primary Specialty (Derived)

| Primary specialty | | Mean number of throat cultures per physician per week | | |
|---|---|---|---|---|
| | | (< 18 yr) Children | (≧ 18 yr) Adults | Total |
| Family practice/ general practice | (N = 140) | 3 (±0.8) | 3 (±1.1) | 6 (±1.6) |
| Internal medicine | (N = 147) | 1 (±0.4) | 2 (±0.7) | 3 (±1.0) |
| Pediatrics | (N = 201) | 15 (±3.4) | 1 (±0.5) | 16 (±3.5) |

Numbers in parentheses (±N) = ±2 Standard error

TABLE 7-9. Use of Throat Culture When Seeing a Patient with Acute Sore Throat, by Specialty

| Primary specialty | Percent always culture | Percent selective culture | Percent never culture | No answer | Percent total (N) |
|---|---|---|---|---|---|
| Family practice/ general practice | 18 | 46 | 36 | (5) | 100 (175) |
| Internal medicine | 16 | 55 | 28 | (2) | 100 (168) |
| Pediatrics | 54 | 42 | 5 | (8) | 100 (224) |
| Weighted totals (All primary care) | 25 | 52 | 23 | | 100 (567) |

*p < .0001 ($\chi^2$=108.15,df=2)
Conservative 95% confidence limits: by specialty, FP/GP±8%, IM±8%, PD±7%, for weighted averages ±5%

pharyngeal exudate, and scarlatiniform rash as clinical signs suggestive of streptococcal infection.

Physical signs rated "decisive" by a majority of practitioners were scarlatiniform rash (72%) and pharyngeal exudate (64%) (Table 7–10). Pediatricians as a group also rated as "decisive" the presence of palatal petechiae (60%) and tender anterior cervical lymph nodes (49%) significantly more often than other primary care practitioners ($p = 0.0065$ and $p = 0.0001$, respectively). The AHA lists headache, fever (usually 101°–104°), and—in children—abdominal pain, nausea, and vomiting, as common presenting symptoms of streptococcal pharyngitis. No symptoms were rated as "decisive" by a majority of primary care practitioners, although feverishness (80%) and chills (72%) were felt to be at least "suggestive" evidence of the need to obtain a throat culture by a majority of physicians (Table 7–11). Pediatricians also rated abdominal pain or vomiting as "suggestive" evidence more often than other primary care physicians ($p = 0.000125$). The desire of the patient (or parent) that a throat culture be obtained was rated "decisive" by 55% of physicians, although significantly fewer pediatricians (33%) rated this item "decisive" (Table 7–12) ($p = 0.0007$). Historic features rated "decisive" by a majority of primary care practitioners were presence of rheumatic heart disease (82%), past history of rheumatic fever (73%), exposure to a case of streptococcal pharyngitis (58%), and a high rate of streptococcal pharyngitis in the community (52%) (Table 7–13).

Of physicians who obtain throat cultures, 74% chose oral penicillin as the preferred form of antibiotic therapy, followed by intramuscular penicillin (11%), ampicillin (9%), erythromycin (6%), and other antibiotics (0.4%) (Table 7–14). No significant differences were noted by specialty.

Antibiotic therapy was started "always" before receiving culture results by 42% of primary care physicians who use throat cultures, and "sometimes," under selected circumstances, by an additional 55% (Table 7–15). Only 3% of physicians indicated that they did not start antibiotic therapy under any circumstances before receiving culture results. Pediatricians (20%) were significantly less likely to start antibiotic therapy "always" compared with internists (43%), or family and general practitioners (52%) ($p < 0.0001$). Of those physicians who started therapy under all or selected circumstances before receiving culture results, 58% ceased therapy if culture results were negative, and 42% completed the planned course of antibiotic therapy despite negative culture results (Table 7–16). Family and general practitioners (45%) were less likely to cease

TABLE 7-10.  Importance of Individual Physical Sign to Physicians Who Selectively Culture

| | Weighted average all primary care | | | |
| Physical sign | Percent decisive | Percent suggestive | Percent not helpful | Percent total (N) |
|---|---|---|---|---|
| Scarlatiniform rash | 72 | 26 | 2 | 100 (260) |
| Pharyngeal exudate | 64 | 34 | 2 | 100 (260) |
| Petechiae of soft palate | 40† | 48 | 12 | 100 (260) |
| Abnormal pharyngeal redness or edema | 33 | 62 | 5 | 100 (260) |
| Tender anterior cervical lymph nodes | 25* | 69 | 6 | 100 (260) |
| Enlarged anterior cervical lymph nodes | 23 | 67 | 10 | 100 (260) |
| Fever | 17 | 66 | 18 | 100 (260) |

†p = .0065      (PD=60%, FP/GP=42%, IM=31%)
*p = .000125    (PD=49%, FP/GP=21%, IM=19%)
Conservative 95% confidence limits for weighted averages ±8%


TABLE 7-11.  Importance of Individual Symptom to Physicians Who Selectively Culture

| | Weighted average all primary care | | | |
| Symptom | Percent decisive | Percent suggestive | Percent not helpful | Percent total (N) |
|---|---|---|---|---|
| Feverishness | 15 | 65 | 20 | 100 (260) |
| Chills | 13 | 59 | 20 | 100 (260) |
| Headache | 5 | 42 | 53 | 100 (260) |
| Abdominal pain or vomiting | 5 | 35* | 60 | 100 (260) |
| Cough or coryza | 2 | 37 | 62 | 100 (260) |

*p = .000125  (PD=60%, FP/GP=32%, IM=29%)
Conservative 95% confidence limits for weighted averages ±8%

TABLE 7-12. Importance of Individual Demographic Feature to Physicians Who Selectively Culture

| Demographic feature | Weighted average all primary care | | | |
| --- | --- | --- | --- | --- |
| | Percent decisive | Percent suggestive | Percent not helpful | Percent total (N) |
| Patient (or parent) desires a culture | 55* | 28 | 17 | 100 (260) |
| Patient is of certain age | 10 | 56 | 34 | 100 (260) |
| Patient is of certain socioeconomic group | 3 | 26 | 71 | 100 (260) |

*p = .0007   (PD=33%, IM=53%, FP/GP=66%)
Conservative 95% confidence limits for weighted averages ±8%

TABLE 7-13. Importance of Individual Historic Feature to Physicians Who Selectively Culture

| Historic feature | Weighted average all primary care | | | |
| --- | --- | --- | --- | --- |
| | Percent decisive | Percent suggestive | Percent not helpful | Percent total (N) |
| Presence of rheumatic heart disease (RHD) | 82 | 15 | 4 | 100 (260) |
| Past history of rheumatic fever (RF) | 73 | 25 | 2 | 100 (260) |
| Exposure to a case of strep pharyngitis | 58* | 40 | 2 | 100 (260) |
| High rate of strep pharyngitis in community | 52 | 47 | 1 | 100 (260) |
| Family history of RF or RHD | 35 | 46 | 19 | 100 (260) |
| Past history of pharyngitis | 11 | 63 | 26 | 100 (260) |

*p = .0130   (PD=43%, FP/GP=58%, IM=65%)
Conservative 95% confidence limits for weighted averages ±8%

TABLE 7-14.  Treatment of Streptococcal Pharyngitis: Preferred Antibiotic of Physicians Who Use Throat Cultures, by Specialty (percentage)

| Antibiotic | Specialty | | | Weighted average all primary care |
| | FP/GP | IM | PD | |
|---|---|---|---|---|
| PO penicillin | 69 | 79 | 76 | 74.3 |
| IM penicillin | 12 | 7 | 13 | 10.5 |
| PO ampicillin | 11 | 8 | 8 | 9.3 |
| PO erythromycin | 7 | 5 | 3 | 5.5 |
| Other | 1 | 0 | 0 | 0.4 |
| Total | 100 | 100 | 100 | 100 (413) |

Conservative 95% confidence limits: by specialty, FP/GP±10%, IM±10%, PD±8%, for weighted averages ±6%

TABLE 7-15.  Antibiotic Therapy of Streptococcal Pharyngitis, by Specialty, for Physicians Who Use Throat Cultures (percentage)

| Do you start antibiotic therapy before receiving culture results? | Specialty | | | Weighted average all primary care |
| | FP/GP | IM | PD | |
|---|---|---|---|---|
| Yes, always | 52 | 43 | 20* | 42 |
| Yes, under selected circumstances | 46 | 54 | 75 | 55 |
| No | 2 | 3 | 4 | 3 |
| Totals | 100 | 100 | 100 | 100 (435) |

*$p < .0001$ ($\chi^2 = 37.821, df = 4$)
Conservative 95% confidence limits: by specialty, FP/GP±10%, IM±10%, PD±7%, for weighted averages ±6%

TABLE 7-16. Antibiotic Therapy of Streptococcal Pharyngitis, by Specialty, for Physicians Who Use Throat Cultures and Who Start Antibiotics Before Receiving Culture Results (percentage)

| Do you cease therapy if the culture is negative? | Specialty | | | Weighted average all primary care |
|---|---|---|---|---|
| | FP/GP | IM | PD | |
| Yes | 45* | 66 | 74 | 58 |
| No | 55 | 34 | 26 | 42 |
| Totals | 100 | 100 | 100 | 100 (376) |

*$p < .0001$ ($\chi^2=25.60$,df=2)

Conservative 95% confidence limits: by specialty, FP/GP±10%, IM±10%, PD±8%, for weighted averages ±6%

antibiotic therapy if culture results were negative, compared with internists (66%), or pediatricians (74%) ($p < 0.0001$). For the group of primary care physicians who use throat cultures, 37% responded that they often did not receive results in time to influence therapy (Table 7–17). Pediatricians (83%) were significantly more likely to receive culture results in time to influence therapy, compared with internists (63%), or family and general practitioners (54%) ($p < 0.0001$).

Throat culture processing time, the average number of days from taking the culture to the physician's awareness of the result, varied by specialty group (Table 7–18). Overall, 38% of primary care physicians received results in ≤ 1 day, an additional 33% in 2 days, an additional 21% in 3 days, and 8% in ≥ 4 days. Pediatricians as a group received results most rapidly, with 65% receiving results in ≤ 1 day, compared with 31% of family and general practitioners, and 27% of internists ($p = 0.0001$).

The method of throat culture most often used by primary care physicians was distributed as follows: presumptive identification by beta-hemolysis (43%); presumptive identification by bacitracin susceptibility (35%); definitive identification of group A strains such as by FA, slide agglutination, or capillary precipitation (20%); and other (2%) (Table 7–19). These data do not separate those who

TABLE 7-17.  Antibiotic Therapy of Streptococcal Pharyngitis, by Specialty, for Physicians Who Use Throat Cultures (percentage)

| Do you often not receive results in time to influence therapy? | Specialty | | | Weighted average all primary care |
|---|---|---|---|---|
| | FP/GP | IM | PD | |
| Yes | 46 | 37 | 17* | 37 |
| No | 54 | 63 | 83 | 63 |
| Totals | 100 | 100 | 100 | 100 (398) |

*p < .0001 ($\chi^2$=27.55,df=2)
Conservative 95% confidence limits: by specialty, FP/GP±10%, IM±10%, PD±8%, for weighted averages ±6%


TABLE 7-18.  Throat Culture Processing Time, by Specialty (percentage)

| Average of days | Specialty | | | Weighted average all primary care |
|---|---|---|---|---|
| | FP/GP | IM | PD | |
| ≦1 | 31 | 27 | 65* | 38 |
| 2 | 32 | 38 | 25 | 33 |
| 3 | 24 | 28 | 6 | 21 |
| ≧4 | 12 | 7 | 4 | 8 |
| Totals | 100 | 100 | 100 | 100 (418) |

*p = .0001, Kruskal-Wallis test
Conservative 95% confidence limits: by specialty, FP/GP±10%, IM±10%, PD±8%, for weighted averages ±6%

TABLE 7-19. Primary Method of Throat Culture, by Specialty, for Physicians Who Use Throat Cultures (percentage)

| Method | Specialty | | | Weighted average all primary care |
|---|---|---|---|---|
| | FP/GP | IM | PD | |
| Throat swab: beta-hemolysis | 41 | 53 | 32 | 43 |
| Throat swab: bacitracin | 31 | 28 | 53* | 35 |
| Throat swab: definitive | 25 | 28 | 12 | 20 |
| Salivary cultures | 0 | 0 | 0 | |
| Gram stain without culture of throat | 0 | 0 | 0 | |
| Other | 2 | 1 | 3 | 2 |
| Totals | 100 | 100 | 100 | 100 (360) |

*$p$ = .00005, ($\chi^2$=25.07,df=4)

Conservative 95% confidence limits: by specialty, FP/GP±12%, IM±13%, PD±8%, for weighted averages ±7%

use bacitracin disks on primary cultures from those who subculture to a second blood agar plate for bacitracin susceptibility. No respondents reported using salivary cultures or gram stain as the primary method. Pediatricians were significantly more likely to employ presumptive identification by bacitracin susceptibility (53%), compared with internists (28%), or family and general practitioners (31%) ($p$ = 0.00005).

Only about one half (236/449) of the primary care physicians who reported using throat cultures responded to questions about the average charges for the primary methods. Therefore, these results can only be considered gross estimates. Average charges by primary method were approximately $9.75 for presumptive identification by beta-hemolysis, $8.45 for presumptive identification by bacitracin susceptibility, and $13.80 for definitive identification (Table 7–20). Paradoxically, the calculated average for beta-hemolysis was greater than for bacitracin susceptibility, although they are not significantly different. These survey results approximate those obtained from a nonrandom survey of selected hospital and private laboratories in metropolitan Atlanta (Table 7–21). Hospital lab charges averaged $12.00 for bacitracin susceptibility and $12.50 for definitive identification. Private lab charges averaged $8.50 for bacitracin susceptibility and $20.00 for definitive identification.

TABLE 7-20. Primary Method of Throat Culture by Specialty and Average Charge (in dollars)

| Method | Average charge for each specialty group | | | Weighted average all primary care |
| | FP/GP | IM | PD | |
|---|---|---|---|---|
| Throat swab: beta-hemolysis | 9.48 | 11.46 | 7.88 | 9.75 |
| Throat swab: bacitracin | 8.12 | 9.44 | 8.29 | 8.45 |
| Throat swab: definitive | 13.60 | 14.63 | 13.00 | 13.80 |
| Totals (N) | (63) | (46) | (127) | (236) |

## DISCUSSION

Our survey results suggest that a substantial proportion (25%) of primary care physicians always use throat cultures in their evaluation of patients with acute sore throat, and 23% manage their patients with acute sore throat without the use of throat cultures. Thus, no universal approach to the role of the throat culture in diagnosis of streptococcal pharyngitis exists among U.S. medical practitioners.

Our survey was not designed to obtain accurate information on the incidence of acute pharyngitis in the United

TABLE 7-21. Throat Culture Methods and Charges for Selected Hospital and Private Laboratories in Metro Atlanta (in dollars)

| Method | Hospital (N=10) lab charges | | Private (N=10) lab charges | |
|---|---|---|---|---|
| | range | avg. | range | avg. |
| Throat swab: presumptive identification by bacitracin susceptibility | 9.00-17.50 | 12.00 (N=3)† | 5.00-15.00 | 8.50 (N=7) |
| Throat swab: definitive identification of group A strains* | 3.00-19.50 | 12.50 (N=6) | -- | 20.00 (N=3) |

†One laboratory charged $35.00 for processing of <u>any</u> culture and was excluded from the analysis

*Such as by FA, slide agglutination or capillary precipitation

States and the frequency of throat culturing. Extrapolating the data from our survey to the universe of 107,201 primary care physicians, this group accounted for approximately 500 million office visits by patients per year in 1982, with the diagnosis of acute pharyngitis made in 80–100 million of these patients. An estimated 28–36 million throat cultures were obtained as a result of these encounters. All of these estimates appear to be inflated when compared with data for only office-based physicians collected by the National Ambulatory Medical Care Survey in 1977–78 [28]. A possible explanation for this degree of overestimation is that our survey was conducted during the peak season for streptococcal pharyngitis and acute respiratory illness, probably leading to overreporting of patient visits and of acute pharyngitis cases by physician respondents. However, a recent comprehensive survey of throat culture practices in Rhode Island found that one throat culture was obtained per 6 persons in that state in 1980 [27], a ratio similar to the estimates derived from our study for the United States.

About half of primary care physicians selectively use throat cultures in their evaluation of patients with acute sore throat. In general, primary care physicians followed existing guidelines [15–24] regarding clinical and epidemiologic factors that suggest streptococcal pharyngitis in deciding whether to obtain a throat culture.

Penicillin was the drug of choice for 85% of the group of primary care physicians who use throat cultures, in keeping with AHA recommendations. However, practitioners greatly preferred oral therapy to the intramuscular penicillin therapy favored by the AHA. The remainder of primary care physicians, with one exception, chose antimicrobial agents that are considered acceptable alternatives.

Notably, 42% of primary care physicians who use throat cultures always start antibiotics before receiving culture results, and an additional 55% do so under selected circumstances. This suggests that the use of throat cultures has a limited role in curtailing exposure of patients to antibiotics and to their possible adverse effects. Pediatricians as a group were less likely to always start antibiotics before receiving culture results than were internists or family and general practitioners. This can be explained, in part, by our finding of significantly shorter throat culture processing time for pediatricians, compared with the other specialty groups.

A surprising finding was that, of those physicians who started antibiotic therapy under all or selected circumstances before receiving culture results, 42% completed the planned course of antibiotic therapy in spite of negative culture results. This finding suggests that many throat cultures have little or no impact either on the decision to begin antibiotic therapy or on the duration of therapy, and would appear to serve only to document the presence or absence of group A streptococci.

Our study provides evidence that opinion is divided among primary care practitioners as to the proper role (if any) of throat cultures in the diagnosis of streptococcal pharyngitis. Their role in primary prevention of acute rheumatic fever has been lessened by the dramatic decline in the incidence and severity of this disease in the United States in the past two decades. We have shown that throat cultures also have a limited role in curtailing widespread use of antibiotics in primary care settings. The fact that throat cultures identify asymptomatic carriers in addition to patients with active streptococcal disease further adds to overtreatment with antibiotics.

Despite these shortcomings, throat cultures are the only accepted, practical tool available to the clinician who desires to make an accurate clinical and laboratory diagnosis of streptococcal pharyngitis before initiating antibiotic therapy. Those clinicians who feel that laboratory diagnosis is desirable may be able to turn to new developments in rapid diagnosis of streptococcal pharyngitis by antigen detection in order to minimize the current widespread practice of initiating antibiotic therapy prior to laboratory confirmation of the presence of the organism.

## REFERENCES

1. Caplan, C. 1979. A case against the use of the throat culture in the management of streptococcal pharyngitis. *J Fam Pract* 8:485–90.
2. Bisno, A. L. 1981. Primary prevention of acute rheumatic fever: quo vadis? *J Lab Clin Med* 98:323–35.
3. Gantz, N. M. 1979. Streptococcal pharyngitis: culture, treat, or both? In *Manual of clinical problems in infectious disease,* 2–5. Gantz, N. M., and R. A. Gleckman ed. Boston: Little Brown.
4. Pantell, R. H. 1977. Cost-effectiveness of pharyngitis management and prevention of rheumatic fever. *Ann Intern Med* 86:497–99.
5. Tompkins, R. K., D. C. Burnes, and W. E. Cable. 1977. An analysis of the cost-effectiveness of pharyngitis management and acute rheumatic fever prevention. *Ann Intern Med* 86:481–92.
6. Bisno, A. L. 1977. Therapeutic strategies for the prevention of rheumatic fever. *Ann Intern Med* 86:494–96.
7. Wannamaker, L. W. 1976. A penicillin shot without culturing the child's throat. *JAMA* 235:913–14.
8. Bisno, A. L. 1979. The diagnosis of streptococcal pharyngitis. *Ann Intern Med* 90:426–28.
9. Morbidity and mortality weekly report—annual summary, 1980. 1981. Atlanta, Georgia: Centers for Disease Control HHS publication (CDC)81–8241.
10. Annegers, J. F, N. L. Pillman, W. H. Weidman, and L. T. Kurland. 1982. Rheumatic fever in Rochester, Minnesota, 1935–1978. *Mayo Clin Proc* 57:753–57.
11. University of Rochester School of Medicine and Monroe County Department of Health. 1978. Infectious Disease Newsletter 23 (25), June 12.
12. Acute rheumatic fever—Texas. 1980. Bureau of Communicable Disease Services, Texas Department of Health. *Texas Morbidity This Week,* September 6.
13. Rhodes P., and H. Jackson. 1975. Rheumatic fever in Colorado—a conquered disease? *JAMA* 234:157–58.
14. Statistical reports, communicable diseases, 1964–1974. Berkeley, Calif: Bureau of Communicable Disease Control.

Department of Public Health, State of California.
15. Kaplan, E. L., A. L. Bisno, W. Derrick et al. 1977. AHA committee report: Prevention of rheumatic fever. *Circulation* 55:S1–4.
16. Honikman, L. H., and B. F. Massell. 1971. Guidelines for the selective use of throat cultures in the diagnosis of streptococcal respiratory infection. *Pediatrics* 48:573–82.
17. Komaroff, A. L. 1978. A management strategy for sore throat. *JAMA* 239:1429–32.
18. Wannamaker, L. W. 1972. Perplexity and precision in the diagnosis of streptococcal pharyngitis. *Am J Dis Child* 124:352–58.
19. Committee Report: Prevention of rheumatic fever. 1965. American Heart Association. *Circulation* 31:948–52.
20. Glezen, W. P., W. A. Clyde, R. J. Senior, C. I. Sheaffer, and F. W. Denny. 1967. Group A streptococci, mycoplasmas, and viruses associated with acute pharyngitis. *JAMA* 202:455–60.
21. Kaplan, E. L., F. H. Top, B. A. Dudding, and L. W. Wannamaker. 1971. Diagnosis of streptococcal pharyngitis: differentiation of active infection from the carrier state in the symptomatic child. *J Infect Dis* 123:490–501.
22. Breese, B. B., and F. A. Disney. 1954. The accuracy of diagnosis of beta streptococcal infections on clinical grounds. *J Pediatr* 44:670–73.
23. Siegel, A. C., E. C. Johnson, and G. H. Stollerman. 1961. Controlled studies of streptococcal pharyngitis in a pediatric population: I. Factors related to the attack rate of rheumatic fever. *New Engl J Med* 265:559–66.
24. Breese, B. B. 1977. A simple scorecard for the tentative diagnosis of streptococcal pharyngitis. *Am J Dis Child* 131:514–17.
25. Wood, R. W., R. K. Tompkins, and B. W. Wolcott. 1980. An efficient strategy for managing acute respiratory illness in adults. *Ann Intern Med* 93:757–63.
26. Gordis, L., L. Desi, and H. R. Schmerler. 1976. Treatment of acute sore throats: a comparison of pediatricians and general physicians. *Pediatrics* 57:422–24.
27. Holmberg, S. D., and G. A. Faich. N.d. Streptococcal pharyngitis and acute rheumatic fever in Rhode Island. Submitted for publication.
28. Cypress, B. K. 1982. Patients' reasons for visiting physicians: national ambulatory care survey, United States, 1977–78. Hyattsville, Maryland: National Center for Health Statistics, DHHS publication (PHS)82–1717. Vital and health statistics; Series 13, No. 56.

29. Moloney, T. W., and D. E. Rogers. 1979. Medical technology—a different view of the contentious debate over costs. *New Engl J Med* 301:1413–19.

30. Bidese, C. M., and D. G. Danais. 1981. Physician characteristics and distribution in the U.S. Chicago: American Medical Association.

# 8

# Methods of Identifying
# Group A Streptococci by Throat Cultures:
# Cost of Materials

*Richard R. Facklam, Ph. D.*

The cost of the materials used for the procedures for the presumptive identification of group A streptococci from throat swabs varies widely and often depends on the volume of material being purchased (Table 8–1). We based our estimates of cost on the purchase of enough supplies to perform a minimum of 100 tests. Estimates of most costs were obtained from at least three different suppliers of materials for each procedure. The estimates shown in Table 8–1 are 1983 costs obtained by telephone contacts or catalogs. Government discounts were not used.

The majority of performance times shown in Table 8–1 were obtained from a 1979 Centers for Disease Control (CDC) publication "Work Time Units—A Diagnostic Workload Measurement Structure for Public Health Laboratories" [1]. This publication gives the time requirements for most of the microbiological procedures used in clinical laboratories. I estimated performance times for all procedures not listed in this manual based on my personal experience with the techniques. The turn-around time in hours is an estimate of the time between the throat swabbing and laboratory result.

The price of swabs varies greatly because the price of individually wrapped fiber-tipped swabs is much less than the swab-transport kits containing transport medium, such as Culturettes or Transwabs, which are in common use. The range of costs for blood agar and selective blood agar plates is dependent upon volume. The average per plate cost of blood agar plates is $0.48 when purchased in lots of

TABLE 8-1. Costs and Time Requirements for Presumptive Identification of Beta-Hemolytic Streptococci from Throat Swabs by Various Methods

| Methods and/or Procedures | Cost of Materials* (dollars) | | | Time | |
|---|---|---|---|---|---|
| | Range | Average | Cumulative Average | Performance (minutes) | Turn around (hours) |
| Swab | 0.07-0.64 | 0.38 | -- | 2-5 | -- |
| Blood agar plate | 0.33-0.65 | 0.48 | 0.86 | 2-3 | 18 |
| Selective BAP | 0.54-0.80 | 0.56 | 1.42 | 2-3 | 18 |
| Bacitracin on primary plates | 0.05-0.09 | 0.07 | 0.93 or 1.49 | 1-2 | 18 |
| Bacitracin subculture | 0.38-0.72 | 0.55 | 1.41 | 2-3 | 42 |
| Presumptive triplate | 0.90-1.50 | 1.10 | 1.96 | 2-3 | 42 |
| Pyrrolidine | -- | 0.55 | 1.41 | 2-3 | 24 |
| Analytab API-205 system | 2.14-2.40 | 2.40 | 3.64 | 5-10 | 44-48 |
| Vitek automated microbiological system | 2.20-3.90 | 3.90 | 5.14 | 5-10 | 44-48 |

*Cost of reusable materials, equipment, and overhead not included. Costs are based on purchase quantities to perform at least 100 tests.

100. The cumulative average cost column lists the average prices of the materials used to that point in the identification procedure; that is, the first cumulative average is the average cost of the swab plus the average cost of the blood agar plate, totaling $0.86. If a selective medium plate is added to the procedure at an additional cost of $0.56, the cumulative average increases to $1.42. Adding a

bacitracin disk to either plate increases the cost an average of $0.07, boosting the cumulative average price to $0.93 and $1.49, respectively.

The turn-around time for determining hemolysis and bacitracin sensitivity of primary cultures is about 18 hours. If subculturing to a second blood agar plate for bacitracin sensitivity is performed, the average cumulative cost is increased to $1.41, and the turn-around time is increased by 24 hours, to 42 hours.

The costs of kits for presumptive tests, such as the triplate, are quite similar. One hundred triplates cost about $1.10 each, and the cumulative cost is $1.96 when the costs of the primary plate and swab are added. Turn-around time for presumptive triplates is the same as bacitracin subculturing, 42 hours.

The pyrrolidine test (PYR) is a new presumptive test for group A streptococci. There are no published data, but results in our laboratory indicate that this test, which requires a 4-hour broth incubation, is specific and sensitive for group A streptococci. When this time is added to the time required to determine the hemolysis from primary cultures, the turn-around time is 20 to 24 hours.

The last two procedures on Table 8-1 are the latest developments in automated identification of streptococci. Both the Analytab API-20S system and the Vitek Automated Microbiological System have included procedures in their systems for identifying group A streptococci. Both are expensive compared to the other presumptive schemes, and both require at least an additional half-day longer than other subculturing procedures. In addition, these procedures require more performance time than other presumptive procedures. We see little or no advantage to these systems for the presumptive differentiation of beta-hemolytic streptococci.

Table 8-2 shows the costs and time requirements for serologic identification of beta-hemolytic streptococci from throat swabs. The cost of complete serologic identification is also included.

Although commercial fluorescent antibody (FA) reagents are available for nongroup A streptococci, they are neither specific nor sensitive enough to be reliable. The average cost of FA identification of group A streptococci is $1.25, and the cumulative cost is $1.63 when the cost of the swab is added. The performance time for all serologic procedures is longer than presumptive testing. The turn-around time for the FA procedure is the shortest of all procedures, about 5 hours, because the FA technique can be applied to mixed cultures after four hours incubation of the swab in

TABLE 8-2.  Costs and Time Requirements for Serologic Identification of
Beta-Hemolytic Streptococci from Throat Swabs

| Methods and/or Procedures | Cost of Materials* (dollars) | | | Time | |
| | Range | Average | Cumulative Average | Performance (minutes) | Turn around (hours) |
| --- | --- | --- | --- | --- | --- |
| Fluorescent antibody | 1.00-2.50 | 1.25 | 1.63 | 5-15 | 5-18 |
| Extraction and Precipitation | | | | | |
| Group A only | 0.36-1.38 | 0.78 | 1.64 | 30-60 | 42 |
| Groups A-G | 1.68-2.70 | 2.10 | 2.96 | 30-60 | 42 |
| Coagglutination and latex agglutination | | | | | |
| Group A only | 0.74-1.25 | 0.95 | 1.81 | 2-8 | 18-24-42 |
| Groups A-G | 2.70-3.94 | 3.08 | 3.94 | 3-10 | 18-24-42 |

*Cost of reusable materials, equipment, and overhead not included.  Costs
are based on purchase quantities to perform at least 100 tests.

broth.  The turn-around time is increased to about 18
hours when the hemolytic results of the culture are required.

The major portion of the costs for serologic identification
of group A streptococci by conventional procedures, that
is, extraction and precipitation, is due to the cost of the
antisera, which is $0.25 per test.  The costs of the ex-
traction procedures vary from $0.08 to $1.10, averaging
$0.78 per group A determination.  When the cost of the
swab and primary blood agar plate is added ($0.86), the
cumulative average cost becomes $1.64.  If the cost of the
antisera for complete identification is included, the average
cost is $2.10 per test and the cumulative costs become
$2.96.  Serologic grouping by extraction and precipitin
testing requires more performance time than any other
procedure and will certainly affect the overall cost of the
determinations.  Turn-around time is at least 42 hours.

Serologic grouping by one of the new slide coagglutination or latex agglutination procedures is a little more

costly than conventional procedures, but both performance time and turn-around time are decreased. These procedures are more specific than presumptive testing and are probably most accurate and convenient to use today.

Table 8–3 lists the sensitivity, specificity, costs, and turn-around time for two newly proposed methods for immediate identification of group A streptococci from throat swabs. The advantage of these procedures is a shortened turn-around time, 60 to 75 minutes for the Abbott Laboratories Enzyme Inhibition Assay method, and 15 to 30 minutes for the nitrous acid extraction-coagglutination procedures proposed by Slifkin [2] and Gerber [3]. The unpublished data for Abbott Laboratories EIA procedure appear very encouraging with high sensitivity and specificity. The two publications regarding the nitrous acid extraction-coagglutination technique reported nearly the same sensitivity and specificity. In both papers, the authors expressed concern over the less than optimal sensitivity of the technique but also felt that the sensitivity could be improved. The development of procedures similar to those listed in Table 8–3 appear to offer a more useful approach for identification of group A streptococci than we have now.

TABLE 8-3.  Proposed Methods For Immediate Identification of Group A Streptococci From Throat Swabs

| Methods | Sensitivity (percent) | Specificity (percent) | Cost (dollars) | Time (minutes) |
|---|---|---|---|---|
| Strep A-EIA (Abbott)* | 96 | 94 | 1.50 | 60-75 |
| Nitrous acid extraction | | | | |
| A. Slifkin[2] | 77 | 96 | 1.50 | 15-30 |
| B. Gerber[3] | 78 | 98 | 0.75 | 15-30 |

*Field testing incomplete

REFERENCES

1.  Centers for Disease Control: A collaboration of the Association of State and Territorial Public Health Laboratory Directors and the Center for Disease Control. 1979. Work Time Units: A Diagnostic Workload Measurement Structure

for Public Health Laboratories.

2. Slifkin, M., and C. M. Gil. 1982. Serogrouping of beta-hemolytic streptococci from throat swabs with nitrous acid extraction and the Phadebact streptococcus test. *J Clin Microbiol* 15:187–89.

3. Gerber, M. A. 1983. Micronitrous Acid Extraction-coagglutination Test for Rapid Diagnosis of Streptococcal Pharyngitis. *J Clin Microbiol* 17:170–71.

# 9

# Diagnosis of Streptococcal Pharyngitis: Non-Culture Methods

*Elia M. Ayoub, M.D.*

Over the past three decades, dependence on clinical criteria for the diagnosis of streptococcal pharyngitis has slowly yielded to the more reliable use of throat cultures. Despite the wide acceptance of this method, many physicians still find this technique less than satisfactory. Objections that have been voiced about the use of throat cultures include the high cost of cultures in certain areas, the high percentage (10%–15%) of false-negative cultures encountered in some clinical settings [1,2] and, above all, the delay in obtaining results. This delay results in difficulties in patient management and administration of therapy. Many patients find it difficult to return for another visit in 24 or 48 hours; or if they can, they object to having to pay for another clinic visit. Some patients will not be treated because they cannot be recalled or are transients. Other patients improve spontaneously, and their parents erroneously conclude that continued medical attention and therapy are no longer necessary.

These drawbacks have stimulated a search for laboratory methods alternative to the throat culture for diagnosing streptococcal pharyngitis (Table 9–1). These methods include nonspecific tests, such as acute phase reactants, and more specific tests for detecting the group A streptococcus or its antigens in tissue and body fluids. The applicability, reliability, and availability of these alternative tests are reviewed in this paper, with particular emphasis on the tests recently developed for rapid identification of the streptococcus and its antigens in pharyngeal secretions.

TABLE 9-1.  Alternatives to Throat Culture

---

A.  Nonspecific tests
    a.  Acute phase reactants: WBC, ESR, CRP
    b.  NBT

B.  Specific tests
    a.  Serological tests for streptococcal antigens
    b.  Tests for detecting streptococcal antigens
        in tissue fluids
        1.  Gram stain
        2.  Fluorescent antibody
        3.  Nitrous acid extraction
        4.  Agglutination technique
        5.  ELISA

---

## NON-SPECIFIC TESTS

### Acute Phase Reactants

The acute phase reactants, particularly the white cell count (WBC), erythrocyte sedimentation rate (ESR), and C-Reactive protein (CRP), are nonspecific indicators of inflammatory reactions in tissues. They are widely used by physicians, often in attempts to differentiate bacterial from nonbacterial infections. It is widely held that acute streptococcal pharyngitis is associated with leukocytosis, elevated ESR, and positive CRP. They cannot be substitutes for throat cultures, but may help to differentiate active infection and the carrier state in pharyngitis patients with a positive culture. Even then, studies suggest that these tests are not very reliable in patients with positive cultures.

In a study by Siegel and his colleagues [3], WBCs greater than $12,000/mm^3$ were present with equal frequency in patients with culture-positive and culture-negative pharyngitis. Similarly, a study [4] of the incidence of elevated ESR (>30 mm/hr) among patients with streptococcal pharyngitis concluded that this test did not help distinguish patients with streptococcal from those with nonstreptococcal pharyngitis. Data on the value of the CRP in streptococcal pharyngitis were provided by Kaplan and Wannamaker [5], who showed that the CRP is positive in 78% of patients with serological evidence of streptococcal pharyngitis. Approximately 50% of patients with pharyngitis and positive throat cultures, but without serological evidence for streptococcal infection, had a positive CRP. Thus, elevated CRP values, as with the WBC and ESR, are present in the majority of patients with acute streptococcal pharyngitis. However, similarly elevated values are also present in a substantial proportion of patients with nonstreptococcal pharyngitis.

## The Nitroblue Tetrazolium Dye Test

Data on the use of the nitroblue tetrazolium dye test (NBT) were reported by Shapera and Matsen [4]. Despite initial hope that this test could effectively differentiate bacterial from nonbacterial infections, results of evaluation of the NBT test in children with streptococcal pharyngitis were disappointing. The percentage of NBT positive cells in peripheral blood of 20 patients with streptococcal pharyngitis was similar to that of 18 patients with nonstreptococcal pharyngitis.

One may sum up the data on the value of acute phase reactants in streptococcal pharyngitis by stating that these tests may be useful in differentiating acute infection from the carrier state in individuals with throat cultures positive for group A streptococcus. However, when used without a throat culture, they are of little value in the diagnosis of streptococcal pharyngitis.

## SPECIFIC TESTS

Specific tests may be divided into two categories, serological tests for antibodies to group A streptococcal antigens, and tests for detecting the group A streptococcus or its antigen(s) in infected tissue.

## Streptococcal Antibody Tests

A number of serological tests are currently available to assay for antibodies to group A streptococcal extracellular products or cellular components [6]. The former category includes the antistreptolysin (ASO), the antistreptokinase, antihyaluronidase, antidesoxyribonuclease B (anti-DNase B), and antinicotinamide adenine dinucleotidase (anti-NADase). Antibodies to cellular antigens include assays for type-specific antibody and antibody to the streptococcal cell wall A carbohydrate. Use of these tests as indicators of antecedent group A streptococcal infection is well-established.

Because a significant rise in these antibodies occurs one to three weeks after acute pharyngitis, streptococcal antibody tests are not useful in the diagnosis of acute streptococcal pharyngitis. Instead, they are used primarily as indicators of antecedent streptococcal infection in the diagnosis of rheumatic fever and glomerulonephritis, and in the differentiation of actual infection and the carrier state in patients with pharyngitis and throat cultures positive for group A streptococcus [7].

## Tests for Detection of Streptococcal Organisms and Antigens in Tissues or Body Fluids

### Gram Stain of Throat Swab

Along with the throat culture, the Gram stain is the earliest laboratory test that enabled identification of the streptococcus as a major pathogen in pharyngitis. This time-honored, simple, expedient and inexpensive technique was rejuvenated recently. Recent studies by Crawford et al. [8] suggest that the Gram stain is associated with 73% sensitivity in diagnosis of streptococcal pharyngitis. However, as in the past, this test suffers from its inability to differentiate group A streptococci from other streptococci normally inhabiting the oropharynx. It would be difficult to envisage a primary use for this test in the diagnosis of streptococcal pharyngitis.

### The Fluorescent Antibody Test

The use of the fluorescent-antibody technique to identify group A streptococci in throat swabs represented the first alternative to throat cultures. The technique most widely used identifies the organisms in broth cultures made directly from throat swabs [9]. The procedure is to incubate the swab in a small volume of culture media (0.5–1 ml of Todd-Hewitt broth) for a period of two to four hours. The sediment is then fixed on a microscopic slide and fluorescein-conjugated group A antiserum applied to the slide. Controls with fluorescein-conjugated normal serum are included. The number of organisms and the intensity of their fluorescence is assessed using a fluorescence microscope.

The degree of correlation between this test and the standard throat culture method has varied. In general, the correlation is good if one includes both positive and negative cultures. However, discrepancies varying from

12% to 63% have been reported [9]. The discrepancies have been primarily due to false-positive reactions with non-group A (that is, groups B, C, and G) streptococci, and to false-negatives in patients whose cultures yield only a few group A colonies.

The reason for the frequent false-positive results remains unknown, although there are at least two possible explanations. They are the use of poorly absorbed antisera, and the presence of Fc receptors on the surface of the streptococcal cell. These problems could be resolved through the use of monoclonal antibodies of high specificity and sensitivity, and by the use of antisera prepared in animal species whose IgG does not bind to streptococcal Fc receptors. However, other drawbacks associated with the use of the fluorescent-antibody technique in endemic situations remain to be resolved. These include the need for expensive equipment, the cumbersome procedure requiring extensive time when a high percentage of negative cultures is expected, and the subjectivity and variability of quantitating fluorescence. It is possible that future technology may overcome these drawbacks, making this technique a reasonable alternative to culture methods.

### Serologic Identification Following Nitrous Acid Extraction

The application of the nitrous acid extraction technique to the rapid identification of small numbers of group A streptococci was reported in 1978 by El Kholy and co-workers [10]. These investigators adapted a microtechnique for extracting group A streptococci from scrapings from tonsillar surfaces, obtained with a blunt plastic spatula. The scrapings are suspended in 20 µl of sodium nitrite, to which glacial acetic acid is added. The extraction proceeds at room temperature for 15 minutes, and the neutralized extract is reacted with streptococcal antiserum using the Lancefield capillary precipitin technique. The test is completed within 30 minutes. Studies of cultures taken from 200 children yielded 34 positive for group A streptococci on blood agar plates. Twenty-eight of 34, or 82%, were identified by the micronitrous extraction technique, and only one of 166 negative cultures gave a false-positive reaction by this technique [10].

### Agglutination Tests

Coagglutination of group A streptococcal cells by antiserum adsorbed to latex particles or to protein A-coated staphy-

lococci has been used to detect the presence of streptococcal cells or solubilized group A carbohydrate antigen in
bacteriological samples. Recently Uchiyama et al. [11]
reported a simple technique for the identification of
streptococcal organisms in throat swabs using a selective
culture medium and a coagglutination method (Phadebact;
Pharmacia Diagnostics, Piscataway, New Jersey). Throat
swabs were placed directly into Todd-Hewitt broth containing trimethoprim-sulfamethoxazole, which allows growth
of group A streptococcus but inhibits other throat flora.
Duplicate swabs were streaked on blood agar plates.
Preincubation of the swabs for four hours allowed detection
of 18 of 19 positives by the coagglutination test, for a
sensitivity of 94%.

An adaptation of this technique and the micronitrous acid
extraction previously described by El Kholy et al. was
reported by Slifkin and Gil [12] and by Gerber [13]. In
this test, the throat swab is first rinsed in a vial containing 0.3 ml distilled water, which is centrifuged; the
sediment is then extracted with nitrous acid for 5 minutes.
The neutralized extract is reacted with the coagglutination
reagents in the Phadebact streptococcus kit, and examined
for agglutination. This procedure yielded a sensitivity of
77% and 78%, respectively, for both investigators, and a
specificity of 98%, when compared to standard blood agar
plate cultures. The majority of false-negatives were
associated with cultures with fewer than 30 colonies. Of
note is that 18 swabs could be processed by this method in
one hour, and the cost per test was approximately $0.25.

These results suggest that the direct coagglutination
technique or the micronitrous extraction followed by a
precipitin or coagglutination test may prove effective
alternatives to throat cultures. This will be true if the
sensitivity of these tests is increased, particularly for
individuals harboring a smaller number of organisms.

### Enzyme-Linked Immunoadsorbent Assay (ELISA) Method

With the proliferation of the use of the ELISA technique as
an immunological tool, it is not surprising to see this
technique adapted for the rapid detection of group A
streptococci in throat swabs. To date, two methods to
detect group A streptococcal antigens in tissue fluids by
the ELISA technique have been described. The first,
reported by Greene and coworkers [14], is a direct technique, called the PELISA test (Figure 9-1). Using a
selective culture medium containing trimethoprim-sulfa-

Figure 9–1. Schematic for PELISA technique used to detect group A streptococcus in throat swabs.

## PELISA TEST

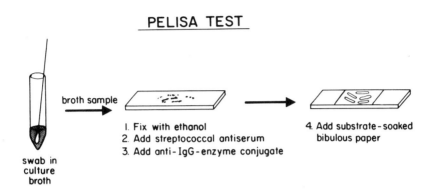

broth sample

1. Fix with ethanol
2. Add streptococcal antiserum
3. Add anti-IgG-enzyme conjugate

4. Add substrate-soaked
   bibulous paper

swab in
culture
broth

methoxazole, a sample of the medium in which the swab was rinsed is plated on a glass slide and fixed with ethanol. Group A streptococcal rabbit antiserum is layered on the slide, washed and dried. Antirabbit IgG, conjugated with horseradish peroxidase, is overlaid on the slide and washed. A strip of substrate-soaked paper (o-diaminobenzene plus hydrogen peroxide) is then placed over the slide. The presence of group A streptococci is revealed by a reaction between the fixed enzyme-conjugated serum and the substrate, producing yellow-orange dots on the bibulous paper. This test takes less than two hours to perform. Recent modifications (Greene, G. R., personal communication) allow reduction of the performance time to 30 minutes. A pilot study on throat swabs from 17 children yielded seven that were positive for group A streptococci on blood agar plate cultures. All swabs from these seven patients were positive by the PELISA technique; two additional PELISA positives were group C streptococci. There were no false-negatives.

Another technique, called the Strep A Enzyme Inhibition Assay (EIA), was described by Knigge, Babb and coworkers [15]. Swabs are incubated in a buffer containing a muralytic enzyme to solubilize group A carbohydrate antigen from streptococcal cell walls. Rabbit group A antiserum is added to the solution, followed by addition of a solid phase that consists of polystyrene beads coated with group A carbohydrate. The reactants are incubated to allow any rabbit antiserum that has *not* been "blocked" by group A carbohydrate solubilized from the swab to bind to the solid-phase A carbohydrate. The solid phase is washed and incubated with goat antirabbit IgG conjugated to horseradish peroxidase, which should react with rabbit IgG that has bound to the solid phase. The latter is then quantitated by incubation with O-phenylenediamine containing hydrogen peroxide. The intensity of the yellow-orange color that develops, which reflects the amount of antibody bound to the coated bead, is read on a spectrophotometer. The percentage of inhibition of color, compared to a positive control, reflects the amount of group A streptococcal antigen solubilized from the throat swab. This test also can be performed in less that two hours. Results of preliminary studies performed on 742 samples collected from patients with pharyngitis yielded 106 positive cultures for group A streptococcus on blood agar plates; 102 of these were positive by the EIA, yielding an agreement of 96% for positive cultures. The overall agreement for both positive and negative samples was 95%.

These findings suggest that both the direct PELISA and the EIA methods show promise for good correlation with conventional culture techniques and have the potential for rapid detection of group A streptococci in throat swabs. The main drawback is that, in addition to the need for a spectrophotometer in the EIA method, these techniques do not differentiate between live and dead organisms and may increase the frequency of identification of pharyngeal carriers of group A streptococci. The question of cost remains to be determined.

CONCLUSION

Throat cultures are currently the mainstay of the diagnosis of streptococcal pharyngitis. The technique is simple, reliable, available, and inexpensive. However, a waiting period of 24–48 hours is required to provide the information needed to allow the physician to decide whether antibiotics should be administered. This primary drawback is the main incentive prompting a search for alternative tests. For any test to qualify as an alternative, it should possess the same attributes as the throat culture, mainly, simplicity, reliability, availability, and low cost, plus the new requisite of expediency. For the practicing physician, expediency means the capacity to provide the necessary information within the shortest time. Utilizing these criteria, tests will be compared to determine which of these, if any, would fulfill these qualifications.

A summary of these tests and their rating with respect to these qualifications is presented in Table 9–2. Based on these criteria, one may conclude tentatively that two techniques—the micronitrous acid extraction with identification by the latex agglutination technique and the ELISA techniques—offer reasonable alternatives to the throat culture as tests for the rapid identification of group A streptococci in patients with pharyngitis. The methods are simple, take two hours or less to perform, show a high degree of specificity, and are inexpensive, with an estimated cost well below one dollar per test. While these tests appear to be promising alternatives to throat cultures, more extensive studies are needed to confirm the value of these tests in the clinical setting of the practicing physician to whom these tests would be most valuable.

TABLE 9-2.  Comparative Value of the Tests for Detecting Streptococcal Antigens in Tissue Fluids

| Test | Simplicity of performance | Sensitivity and specificity | Reagent availability | Time performance/ results | Cost/Unit |
|------|---------------------------|-----------------------------|----------------------|---------------------------|-----------|
| 1. Fluorescent antibody | 4 | 2 | 3 | 3 | 1 |
| 2. Coagglutination | 1 | 3 | 2 | 3 | 1 |
| 3. Nitrous acid extraction: | | | | | |
|    a. Precipitin | 3 | 2 | 2 | 1 | 1 |
|    b. Coagglutination | 2 | 2 | 2 | 1 | 1 |
| 4. ELISA: | | | | | |
|    a. PELISA | 2 | 1 | 2 | 2 | 2 |
|    b. EIA | 2 | 1 | 2 | 2 | 2 |

Grading Scale: 1 = most acceptable; 4 = least acceptable

110

# REFERENCES

1.  Taranta, A., and M. D. Moody. 1971. Diagnosis of streptococcal pharyngitis and rheumatic fever. *Ped Clin North Am* 18:125.

2.  Battle, C. V., and L. A. Glasgow. 1971. Reliability of bacteriologic identification of beta-hemolytic streptococci in private offices. *Am J Dis Child* 122:134.

3.  Siegel, A. C., E. E. Johnson, and G. H. Stollerman. 1961. Controlled studies of streptococcal pharyngitis in a pediatric population. I. Factors related to the attack rate of rheumatic fever. *New Engl J Med* 265:559.

4.  Shapera, R. M., and J. M. Matsen. 1973. Nitroblue tetrazolium dye reduction by neutrophils from patients with streptococcal pharyngitis. *Pediatrics* 51:284.

5.  Kaplan, E. L., and L. W. Wannamaker. 1977. C-reactive protein in streptococcal pharyngitis. *Pediatrics* 60:28.

6.  Ayoub, E. M. 1982. Streptococcal antibody tests in rheumatic fever. *Clin Immunol Newsletter* 3:107.

7.  Kaplan, E. L., F. H. Top, Jr., B. A. Dudding, and L. W. Wannamaker. 1971. Diagnosis of streptococcal pharyngitis: The problem of differentiating active infection from the carrier state in the symptomatic child. *J Infect Dis* 123:490.

8.  Crawford, G., F. Brancata, and K. K. Holmes. 1979. Streptococcal pharyngitis: diagnosis by Gram stain. *Ann Intern Med* 90:293.

9.  Ayoub, E. M., and L. W. Wannamaker. 1964. Identification of group A streptococci: Evaluation of the use of the fluorescent-antibody technique. *JAMA* 187:908.

10.  El Kholy. A., R. Facklam, G. Sabri, and J. Rotta. 1978. Serologic identification of group A streptococci from throat scrapings before culture. *J Clin Microbiol* 8:725.

11.  Uchiyama, N., G. Greene, J. Carruthus, and E. Mendoza. 1982. Early detection of group A strep (GAS) in acute pharyngitis using Phadebact. Presented at the meeting of the Lancefield Society, Miami, Florida.

12.  Slifkin, M., and G. M. Gil. 1982. Serogrouping of beta-hemolytic streptococci from throat swabs with nitrous acid extraction and the Phadebact streptococcus test. *J Clin Microbiol* 15:187.

13.  Gerber, M. A. 1982. Micronitrous acid extraction-coagglutination test for rapid diagnosis of streptococcal pharyngitis. (Abstract). Program and Abstracts of the 22nd Interscience Conference on Antimicrobial and Chemotherapy (4–6 October), 168.

14.  Greene, G. R., K. Brillhart, and N. Uchiyama.

1982. Rapid detection of group A strep in the pharynx by paper enzyme-linked immunoadsorbent assay. (Abstract). Program and Abstracts of the 22nd Interscience Conference on Antimicrobial Agents and Chemotherapy (4–6 October), 168.

15. Knigge, K., J. Babb, K. Ancell, S. Hurli, and J. Firca. Enzyme Immunoassay for the detection of group A streptococci. Personal communication.

# 10

# Diagnosis of Pharyngitis

## Discussion

### CLINICAL PREDICTION OF THE DIAGNOSIS OF STREP THROAT

DR. SANFORD: Has anybody here tried to confirm Breese's observations or apply them using other scoring systems?

DR. TOMPKINS: In a number of populations, both adults and children, we have used many of Breese's original variables as predictors. We have been unable to confirm the high predictability rate that he observed in any of the populations, using a variety of kinds of providers, both board-certified pediatricians, internists, and nonphysician practitioners.

I have been unable on a statistical basis to come up with as high a predictability rate for any of the criteria that they used, and I am not sure what the differences are. Some of Breese's original studies didn't specify very clearly the population groups they were studying, so it was hard to compare what they did to what we did.

All of our studies were based upon an entry symptom, namely, sore throat, and excluded certain age groups. For instance, the kids are all over two years old. We collected a well-defined data base on all patients, which included not only symptoms and physical findings, but also laboratory data. In many cases, we actually did joint blinded simultaneous examinations by two providers to look at the reproducibility of the various findings.

From the data that we collected on very large numbers of patients, we constructed a variety of strategies, protocols, scoring indices—call them what you will—using the positive throat culture for streptococci as the end point.

We did reasonably well in predicting positive throat cultures in a very small percentage of the patients and reasonably well in predicting negative throat cultures in a very high percentage of the patients. This was related to the fact that most patients had negative cultures.

However, there was a huge middle group, and at either end of it, we were not nearly as good as Breese and Disney's group's predictions. The other thing that became clear as we studied more and more populations was that there are many algorithms or scoring systems that can be developed. You can sort of tailor them not only to the population and the providers, but also to what your outcome index is. We have constructed 30 or 40 different algorithms for different age groups, depending on what we wanted to do. If we wanted to reduce the use of throat cultures, we had one set of algorithms; if we wanted to triage patients over the phone, we had an algorithm to get them to the doctor's office or get them to the pharmacy.

The algorithms were not only specific for those outcomes but, although they all have certain common characteristics, they also varied somewhat by population and by group.

DR. WANNAMAKER: What differences did you find between school-aged children and adults?

DR. TOMPKINS: One of the most critical things was, as you pointed out in your analysis, that there was nothing that really stood out in either age group as being terribly important as a single predictor. A combination of signs and symptoms was necessary. The algorithms that we developed for kids were a little bit different from those for adults, but not tremendously so.

I can't answer your question specifically as to whether or not there was one thing that distinguished clearly between the two groups.

DR. WANNAMAKER: Did you have a higher predictability in adults than school-aged children?

DR. TOMPKINS: No, not really, when we corrected for the incidence of positive streptococcal cultures. In all of the populations that we have looked at, the incidence of positive cultures in adults presenting with sore throats is 8%–10% and in kids 18%–20%. This relates to data from 40,000 to 50,000 patients with upper respiratory illnesses, about 60% of whom have sore throats. These patients were not concentrated in strictly urban or inner-city areas, but represent a fairly diffuse population group.

DR. DILLON: Dr. Tompkins, who made your observations in the clinical assessment of patients that you studied à la Breese and associates?

DR. TOMPKINS: We have had a series of three study groups and many other groups that I won't discuss. The three study groups included one pediatric clinic population in which observations were made by physicians' assistants and staff pediatricians; in a certain specified subset of cases, they were made blindly and jointly on the same patients.

There were two groups of adults. One was in an army medical clinic in which board-certified internists examined a subset of patients jointly and blindly with physicians' assistants, but the majority were examined by physicians' assistants alone. There was a third group, which was basically an adult general medical clinic in an HMO in Nashua, New Hampshire, in which the observations were made entirely by physicians' assistants with confirmation in a less rigorous way by the internists who ran the clinic.

In addition the preliminary studies that led to setting up these much larger studies were done by my colleagues and myself. All observations were made by my colleagues and myself, all either internists on the faculty or in a post-residency fellowship. But the majority of the studies are with nonphysician observers.

However, the interesting thing is that the numbers don't change much when you compare those of internists, for instance, to those of the physicians' assistants. Reproducibility between physicians and between physicians' assistants and the internists is basically indistinguishable.

DR. DILLON: In our own experience in the pediatric outpatient setting, when he was the pediatric outpatient doctor, Warren Derrick used a patient data check sheet and cultures very much like Breese's group, and he found that predictability of streptococcal pharyngitis correlated with a number of things that Dr. Wannamaker has mentioned. Certain seasons of the year certainly would influence this, but the statistically significant observation was that children with acute exudative pharyngitis plus tender lymph nodes in whom throat cultures revealed large numbers of group A streptococci were those most often predicted by the house officer as likely having streptococcal disease. There was a very significant predictable association. If you got away from the group with strongly positive cultures and looked then only at the combination of tender nodes and exudative pharyngitis in patients with one to two plus cultures, the predictability was still greater that they had strep than nonstrep, but the significance tailed off. Conversely, the predictability was least in children who presented with sore throat without either of those findings; the majority of those patients would have smaller numbers of strep or be in the negative-culture group.

DR. TOMPKINS: I would like to point out, Dr. Dillon, a problem with the kind of analysis that you are making.

It's likely that you are able on the basis of clinical findings to improve your predictive accuracy over what the initial guess would be. For instance, in a population of adults with sore throats who have an overall incidence of about 10% positive streptococcal cultures, by using data appropriately in a statistical fashion and with whatever scoring system you use, we can get to a point where we can select out a high risk group with 25%–30% positive throat culture rates. It's really hard to do much better unless you become very, very exclusive and limit the numbers tremendously. A pediatric population may have an overall 20%–30% initial rate. You can probably take it up to 50%–60% using similar kinds of techniques.

However, as you increase the initial incidence of positive streptococcal cultures in your population, by whatever means, you seem to be getting better and better in your predictive ability but are basically doubling it, based upon what your guess would be at the start by all your clinical refinements. I wonder if a lot of the differences that we see between Dr. Breese's original work and ours are based upon a selection of the population at the beginning of the study. Perhaps some of the comments about the ability to predict strep throat during epidemics of other diseases presenting with pharyngitis are really related to the fact that you are getting a dilution effect, not to the fact that your predictability is changing a great deal.

DR. DILLON: I'm not sure how important it is that we are able to make this prediction, if you put it in the perspective of what we have been doing over many years—the concept that it is legitimate to take the culture and then wait for therapy. I think you are making some observations that are highly important. The observations of Warren Derrick were made within the same framework that the teaching program was instituted. Patients with even minimal respiratory complaints are likely to be cultured in such a setting, so one does add to the numbers.

I'm not trying to make a case for predictability, but that in a situation where consistent observations in a consistent culture program are made over a period of time, these were the factors that correlated.

DR. TOMPKINS: I agree with you if the word "consistent" is used. But I think the issue here is consistency.

One of the problems with these kinds of observations is that they are not really consistent when you analyze the data we gathered and how many patients actually get cultured. My only point is that the consistency of data in housestaff programs is less than ideal. One finds that not all patients get throat cultures, not all have the same kinds of clinical information collected, and information is not collected in the same way, so that making statements about ability to predict is a little bit dangerous.

I would urge that in discussing clinical strategies like algorithms or scoring systems that we really have to limit analysis or discussion to those studies in which a standardized data base, including throat culture and whatever other tests are thought appropriate, have been collected on everybody who has met the criteria for the study, to avoid those in which less rigorous approaches have been used.

DR. DILLON: I completely agree with you. One of the reasons that I particularly like Derrick's data is that he saw patients himself and made reconfirming observations.

DR. SHULMAN: Is there a difference between Breese's studies and Derrick's studies in which all patients with respiratory complaints were included, and your studies, Dr. Tompkins, in that the entry point is a complaint of sore throat?

DR. TOMPKINS: Actually, that was a subset of a larger study in which all data for respiratory complaints were entered. We have analyzed the total population and found that that was not really worthwhile doing. In our populations, about 60% of the patients with respiratory complaints also had a symptom of sore throat.

We did a follow-up of all patients that were involved in our studies up to two months after they had originally been seen. In the almost 5,000 adult patients and the 2,000–3,000 pediatric patients we studied, we saw absolutely no cases of acute rheumatic fever, whether patients were treated or not. Although we looked for rheumatic fever as an outcome variable, the last time I saw a case was with Dr. Rammelkamp—or maybe it was with Dr. Mortimer—back in housestaff training days.

DR. PANTELL: I want to comment on the predictivity of the data that you presented from Breese. In one table he had a positive predictivity of 82%–84%, which looks pretty good. However, we need to consider the base rate of positivity which for that table was 58% of cultures. Increasing from 58% to the mid-80s isn't quite as impressive as might first seem. It's important to consider what diagnosticity we will get in situations with a 15% positive culture rate. There is really no way to extrapolate from data derived from 40%–50% prevalence. In a study in Ohio in the last several years, again in school-aged children, they were able to increase from 40% to about 80% predictivity, but for most of us dealing with 15% positivity, the predictivity is much, much lower because the prevalence is so much lower.

DR. HOUSER: By Bayesian analysis, given the sensitivity and specificity of the data, you can determine predictability with a 15% or any other prevalence rate.

DR. PANTELL: I'm not sure we really can from this type of clinical data. It's certainly true that if we have a single diagnostic test or measurement and you know sensitivity and you know specificity, you know prevalence.

## THE VALUE OF NASAL CULTURES FOR STREPTOCOCCI

DR. DENNY: Lew, you did not mention either nasal or nasopharyngeal cultures. The old data from Hamburger's studies showed that the nasal culture was predictive of acute infection. What is the status of nose and nasopharyngeal cultures in 1983, particularly with reference to the age of the patient?

DR. WANNAMAKER: I don't know whether I can answer your question or not. In our initial attempts to look at children in Minnesota, we were taking nose and throat cultures, and we soon gave them up because we found so few positive nose cultures. We didn't take nasopharyngeal cultures.

DR. DENNY: So nasal cultures don't seem to be important in children?

DR. WANNAMAKER: I don't think so. One of the problems, as I see it, with Hamburger's and Erman's studies was that they were really pretty selective in what they were looking for. I think our studies from Warren Air Force Base suggested that those patients who had positive nose cultures were more likely to spread the organism, but the percentage with positive nose cultures was not very high. Even with acute infections they were only about a fifth to a third of the patients, as I recall.

DR. DENNY: Does the streptococcus grow in the nasopharynx?

DR. WANNAMAKER: I think it does in a young infant. It's uncommon in adults, and when you find it in adults, it's frequently a sign of sinusitis. But we didn't find it very useful in trying to make a diagnosis of strep infection in children in Minnesota.

DR. SHULMAN: Does anyone else have experience with

nasal or nasopharyngeal cultures?

DR. HOUSER: I am trying to recall the Warren data. When there were "transitory acquisitions," weren't those more likely to be found in the nose than in the throat?

DR. WANNAMAKER: Yes. They were very common, but I wouldn't call those infections.

DR. HOUSER: No, but the question was related to reproducibility in the nose.

## THE ROLE OF OTHER AGENTS IN ACUTE PHARYNGITIS

DR. BISNO: Lewis, what is your feeling about the role of non-group A strepococci in sporadic cases of pharyngitis? In the rheumatic fever prophylaxis populations that we cultured over the years, there is an awfully high carriage rate of Group Cs, Gs, and other non-As. We are all very familiar with the reported instances of food-borne epidemics of non-A pharyngitis.

Does anyone have a feeling about the role, if any, of these non-group As, particularly Cs and Gs, as cause of sporadic pharyngitis?

DR. WANNAMAKER: In our experience in Minnesota, they are pretty uncommon. But if one looks at some of the data from Egypt and the African countries, they seem to be pretty common, at least in terms of acquisition. Some indicate that they are associated with clinical findings. And there is some evidence to indicate, as least in the Egyptian studies, that they are associated with an antibody response. It may depend on the population group. There was some indication from the Nashville studies that Cs and Gs were increasing, but I don't think that really continued in subsequent surveys in those school populations.

DR. DENNY: That was never very impressive in the studies we did in Nashville. But in our short-term studies in college students several years ago, non-group As, specifically groups C and G, were equal to group A as causes of antibody-responsive pharyngitis.

DR. KOMAROFF: In our study of 700 adults in the late 1970s in New England, we found equivalent isolation rates of group A and non-group A strep. Only about 5% of the latter were associated with antibody rises, in contrast to roughly 35% of the group A strep. In a recent ICAAC abstract, the Syracuse Health Service reported about a 15% isolation rate of non-group A strep in pharyngitis, compared to 1% to 2% in the control group of patients presenting with nonrespiratory infections at the same time. This was a significant difference. Interestingly, there was not a significant difference in group A strep isolation rates when pharyngitis patients were contrasted to nonpharyngitis controls. I have the impression from our data that non-group A strep pharyngitis is a clinical entity in young adults. Whether treating it will matter is obviously debatable.

DR. AYOUB: I wonder how we can come to a conclusion about the role of non-group A strep infection when we have no specific tests that allow us to come to any conclusions about whether there is infection or carriage. As I recall, in the 1960s when we did fluorescent antibody studies on University of Minnesota students, the rate of non-group As was almost as frequent as group A in those with pharyngitis. Until we get specific tests, I think it would be futile to argue about the role of this organism in pharyngitis.

DR. DILLON: Dr. Wannamaker's slide incited a comment about the prevalence of other agents in the community. When we began to get data on influenza viruses in children, we were able to show that in January and early February of several consecutive years when influenza was at a peak, children presenting in the clinic with acute sore throat and fever without exudate had negative cultures. The streptococcus seems to disappear when the influenza virus is in the community, and it reappears when this agent is not around. If you look at children with sore throat at the height of a flu epidemic, you are not going to find a streptococcus and you can predict with almost 100% accuracy that they don't have this disease.

DR. WANNAMAKER: I don't think that's our experience at Warren Air Force Base with young adults. During several flu epidemics, the rate of streptococcal infection stayed constant throughout striking peaks of influenza. We had more streptococcal pneumonia, but not streptococcal pharyngitis.

DR. SHULMAN: Are you saying that during those times the proportion of symptomatic patients who had strep fell, but the absolute numbers remained constant?

DR. WANNAMAKER: Yes, the ones who met the criteria we were using all along.

DR. DENNY: I don't believe we have any data at all on group A streptococcus and what it does during viral epidemics. It's true that when one looks at other agents in a community, there is to a certain extent mutual exclusiveness of organisms. In other words, whenever influenza comes in, other viruses seem to disappear. I don't believe we have any data on that with respect to streptococci.

DR. STOLLERMAN: There are data like that. The Great Lakes group studied adenovirus and flu in the recruit population years ago and showed a mutually exclusive epidemiology for influenzae, adenovirus, and streptococci. That was quite a strong report, but I don't think it ever received the attention it deserved.

DR. DAVIS: I would like to raise some interesting possibilities. If you are talking about nonviral agents, they could colonize a mucous membrane for a longer period. I think the whole issue of seasonality might be obscured because other agents could persist for as long as the streptococcus. That might then affect one's ability to be colonized with certain kinds of strep.

We have seen a lot of mycoplasma in Wisconsin for the last couple of years, much more than had ever been described diagnostically in the state. This is from looking at trends at two different laboratories within the state.

DR. DENNY: This is fascinating to me, because we are beginning to examine whether positive throat cultures for pneumococci are predictive of certain types of respiratory disease. In a preliminary way, it looks as though the percentage of influenza patients presenting with lower respiratory tract infection who have pneumococci is very low, which is in contradistinction to what we have been led to believe with influenza. So there might well be something to the exclusivity of these organisms.

DR. WATANAKUNAKORN: In our hospital, we have seen a number of young adults with sore throat whose throat cultures grew large numbers of *Hemophilus influenzae*. Is there an entity of hemophilus pharyngitis? What do you do with it?

DR. SHULMAN: A major medical textbook includes hemophilus as a cause of pharyngitis, but I would like to hear from this group. I assume we are talking about untypeable hemophilus.

DR. SCHWARTZ: We have a paper in press in *Pediatrics* on the prevalence of *H. influenzae* in well children, in children who had just finished a course of amoxicillin for otitis, and in children with purulent nasopharyngitis. We did paired cultures of the nasopharynx and the throat. Establishing an etiologic link between pharyngitis and *H. influenzae* is difficult because 60% of well children have *H. influenzae* in their throats. Most are nontypeable; of 249 isolates, only six were type b. Other typing wasn't performed. It would be hard to prove unless one could show that those with nasopharyngitis or pharyngitis had an antibody response against nontypeable *H. influenzae*. The children with purulent nasopharyngitis had no higher incidence of hemophilus than the healthy children. Most of these children were between six months and three years of age. We used selective media, chocolate agar with 12 U/mL of bacitracin.

DR. WASHINGTON: Some years ago, Rose studied the role of *H. influenzae* in pharyngitis because pediatricians believed it was important. She examined 490 children with upper respiratory illness and 490 children without upper respiratory disease. The only organisms for which there was any statistically significant difference were group A strep and viruses. There was no significant difference in *H. influenzae* or non-group A beta-hemolytic strep.

DR. BISNO: I would like to caution that because there is a tremendous carriage rate of *H. influenzae* doesn't mean there are not cases of *H. influenzae* pharyngitis. Certainly we never considered *H. influenzae* a major pathogen in adults 20 years ago. It was so rare that anyone who saw a case of *H. influenzae* meningitis in adults would rush to publish it, but now there is much literature on significant *H. influenzae* infections in adults.

DR. HILL: In addition, you have to realize that a lot of otitis media is caused by nontypeable *H. influenzae*, so we really can't consider it totally nonpathogenic.

DR. KOMAROFF: In our studies with Norden using both isolation rates and serologic studies, we found rates of only 1% to 2% of *H. influenzae* in young adults. It was very questionable whether it was a pathogen. Nevertheless, especially in the fall of 1982, I saw four or five pharyngitis patients within two months who had heavy growth of *H. influenzae* and nothing else. They had penicillin-unresponsive disease that improved dramatically within 12 to 24 hours when they were switched to ampicillin.

I would like to mention some unpublished data that suggest that other nonstreptococcal organisms may play a role in pharyngitis. We studied adults in the late 1970s in New England, looking initially at the incidence of streptococcal and viral pharyngitis. Subsequently, in a group of about 150 adult patients, we looked for other potentially treatable organisms serologically. The streptococcal rate was 9%. In 3% there were fourfold rises in antibody to *Legionella* or *Hemophilus*, and in 15% titers to *Legionella* and *Hemophilus* were greater than 1:128. Mycoplasmal serology showed fourfold rises in 11% and high single titers in others. We also found fourfold rises in antibody to *Chlamydia trachomatis* in 21% of the patients. These are only retrospective serologic data, and we had not attempted to obtain cultures prospectively. However, we are attempting to pursue this with better cultures and a randomized treatment trial with erythromycin. I hope we don't find erythromycin very effective because of the concerns from the Japanese experience and its gastrointestinal toxicity. But maybe there are other infectious agents besides group A streptococcus that we should consider.

## BACTERIOLOGIC DIAGNOSIS OF STREP PHARYNGITIS

DR. WASHINGTON: We recently extended the Murray studies in our laboratory from several years ago, evaluating once more the atmosphere of incubation with about 2,000 cultures. The group A isolation rates at 24 hours on sheep blood agar were approximately 16% aerobically and 13% anaerobically. At 48 hours they were 18% and 17%, respectively, so they evened out roughly. We resubstantiated the earlier studies.

DR. BISNO: Does that include $CO_2$?

DR. WASHINGTON: Yes, $CO_2$ at 24 hours yielded 11.6% and at 48 hours 15.6%, so it was still the least sensitive. However, for non-group A beta-hemolytic strep, the percentages in air and $CO_2$ and anaerobically were 11.9%, 13.3%, and 29.4%, respectively. Again anaerobic conditions increased recovery of non-group A strep.

DR. SCHWARTZ: Since October 1982, for every symptomatic child who had a throat culture taken, I have had duplicate cultures taken with two swabs plated on sheep blood agar. Cultures were saved until the end of the morning or afternoon shift, then one of each pair was placed in an anaerobe jar and the other in a regular incubator. Both were incubated at 37° C. To date, we have almost 1,300 paired cultures.

Every discrepant culture was grouped for A and G. A data sheet was filled out with patients' symptoms; telephone calls were made daily until the symptoms were gone; and most importantly, patients were asked to come in initially and then three weeks later for blood for streptozyme and exoenzyme serology.

So far, our findings are markedly different from Dr. Washington's. There were 245 positive (>2+) throat cultures, all of which were bacitracin sensitive and group A, for an overall 18% rate by the aerobic technique. However, 324 were positive anaerobically, and 80% of those were at least 3+. Only two cultures positive aerobically didn't grow in the anaerobe jar, both being only 2+. Seventy-nine group A streps (>2+) were positive in the anaerobe jar, but not by the aerobic technique.

So far we have 17 paired serologic titers from day 1 and after three weeks; four of 17 seroconverted, so we are not dealing only with carriers. I'm firmly convinced that the anaerobic technique is superior. That was not my bias when I began the study, by the way.

DR. GERBER: Did you use subsurface stabbing on the aerobic plates?

DR. SCHWARTZ: Yes, we always do.

To clarify our procedure, plates are put into the anaerobe jar three times a day. If a culture is taken at 9 a.m., it stays out until noon, when it's put into the jar. We swab and streak the plates immediately and place an A disk on the primary plate. The anaerobic and aerobic plates are put into the incubator three times a day. One interesting finding is that we subcultured those cultures that grew only anaerobically to see if they would grow aerobically. Eighty percent of them grew, but didn't produce beta-hemolysins.

DR. KAPLAN: What kind of plates do you use?

DR. SCHWARTZ: Five percent sheep blood agar.

DR. MORTIMER: Having once gotten caught on this, I would like to point out that a possible explanation for the discrepancies in these studies might be systematic errors that creep in, such as the unintentional bias of the technician streaking a plate.

DR. FACKLAM: I have reviewed numerous manuscripts on differences in isolation rates of group A strep, and I cannot explain the differences. There is no way unless there is technician bias.

DR. WASHINGTON: How often do you see a group A streptococcus that doesn't produce hemolysis?

DR. FACKLAM: Very rarely. I think I have about 15 strains collected over 15 years.

DR. DENNY: Since we usually recognize group A streptococci by their hemolysis, is your statement that you have seen only a handful over the years correct? Would you have recognized group A streptococci if they were non-hemolytic?

DR. FACKLAM: You have to go back to some old fluorescent antibody studies, especially in Connecticut, where controls were done. Once a year, 400 consecutive swabs were studied independently of hemolysis on plates. After five years, they stopped doing this because they never found a discrepancy.

DR. SANFORD: Most of the time we assume that the agar base we use is reasonably consistent, even though most agar is nothing but piles of seaweed. There may well be considerable differences, even though this is theoretically an inert base.

DR. FACKLAM: There have been two outbreaks of nonhemolytic group A strep in this country—the Lowrey Air

Force Base strain, which was rheumatogenic, and another outbreak of wound infections—but the strains were indeed nonhemolytic on the surface. There was no problem because they were isolating pure cultures.

DR. HOUSER: At Lowrey there was no rheumatic fever. They had excellent surveillance and treatment and suddenly had an outbreak of rheumatic fever on the base. These people had negative cultures. They looked back and found that nonhemolytic strep were present and identified them as group A.

DR. DILLON: I want to amplify what Dr. Sanford said. The type 43 strain didn't grow, because it didn't have yeast extract in the agar base. Too little attention has been paid to quality of media. We have to make huge numbers of blood agar plates because of studies, and we find a lot of variation of individual base lots. When Maxted visited Dr. Wannamaker's laboratory, he demonstrated how markedly different colonial morphology and degree of hemolysis were, depending on the blood agar base used to prepare the medium. In commercial media available in our community, there is a lot of variation, sometimes all or none in the sense of discrepant results.

DR. WANNAMAKER: I think there is a lot of difference in the way various strains behave when cultured in various ways. Dr. Schwartz, I would be interested to know if you had mostly one strain in your population. I suppose you didn't do any typing.

DR. SCHWARTZ: I did in previous years, and they were different strains.

DR. WANNAMAKER: We have had runs when there clearly was a difference between aerobic and anaerobic recovery rates and other times when there didn't seem to be. Did you do stabs in your aerobic plates?

DR. SCHWARTZ: Yes.

DR. WANNAMAKER: And you had the impression that they were not helpful?

DR. SCHWARTZ: No, I didn't say that. If a stab was positive, then that plate would be considered positive. But I would say fewer than 5% of aerobically incubated plates were stab positive without beta-hemolytic colonies on the surface. It does help, but it's only about 5%.

DR. BISNO: Of the six studies you reviewed, three showed that anaerobic incubation was superior to aerobic in isolation of group A. Of the other three, I think it was Dr. Washington's in which there was no significant difference. Were there any studies in which anaerobic incubation had an unfavorable effect?

DR. GERBER: No.

DR. BISNO: So really the issue is whether you want to pick up all the non-group As you will get anaerobically. There is no study in the literature that indicates that anaerobic incubation is deleterious, and three of six studies indicate that it's actually beneficial in isolating group As.

DR. GERBER: That's right. But even in the studies that showed an increased yield of group A, there was also an increased yield of non-group A, which resulted in more subculturing and potentially more false-positives.

DR. HOUSER: All studies are not equal. It's not necessary in trying to solve a problem to add up the studies and put them on one side or the other, but rather to divide them according to what you are looking for. This gets back to what Dr. Dillon was saying—if you use rigorous standards you may change the results. But is the purpose to use standards that duplicate office practice or standards that can be duplicated only in a research laboratory? I suggest that the one that's done in the office using a commercial medium might be more relevant.

DR. HILL: How practical is it to use anaerobic isolation techniques in the practitioner's office?

DR. KAPLAN: Ten or 12 years ago, Stillerman and Moody did a similar study. One of the conclusions was that anaerobic incubation allowed them to read their cultures for hemolysis earlier. Anaerobic incubation allowed them to read their plates as positive as early as six or eight hours.

DR. GERBER: Dr. Washington's data showed no difference at 24 or 48 hours; I don't recall any studies that looked at earlier intervals.

DR. KAPLAN: In the study by Ederer that you quoted, were the data based on pure cultures or primary plates?

DR. GERBER: They were all subcultures.

DR. KAPLAN: When you talk about the 96%, are you talking about pure strep?

DR. GERBER: That's right.

DR. DAJANI: I understand that you are recommending that the 10 mm zone for bacitracin not be adhered to. You said that would increase sensitivity. What does it do to specificity?

DR. GERBER: There is some evidence that it actually decreased specificity. The only study that addressed this was the one by Ederer. Sensitivity dropped from 100% to 96% when they used the zone size. There is no comment on what that did to specificity.

DR. DAJANI: My concern is that if you don't adhere to 10 mm, you are going to read too many non-group As as group As.

DR. GERBER: That's less of an error than the other

way. I would rather have the test be less specific and more sensitive.

DR. FACKLAM: I don't see how you can start requiring a specific zone size on something that doesn't have a standard inoculum or standard media or a standard atmosphere. I think it's just not feasible.

DR. BALTIMORE: You are quoting vastly different rates using different culture techniques, some using selective media and several using nonselective media. We need data comparing sequential cultures in the same patient, using selective media and nonselective media to help to distinguish why these rates are so different.

## SURVEY OF PHYSICAN PRACTICES

DR. MORTIMER: In terms of the physician survey, it probably belabors the obvious to say that the absolute percentages probably don't mean much because of the response rate. However, the relative proportions of the responses of different physicians probably do mean something.

DR. HILL: What percentage of throat cultures are done in the physician's office as opposed to in a true microbiology laboratory?

DR. COCHI: We have these data but, unfortunately, I don't have the numbers with me at this time.

DR. SHULMAN: Certainly, the decreased turnaround time reported by pediatricians suggests that they are doing cultures in their offices for the most part.

DR. HOUSER: Is the use of antibiotics any different among physicians who do not culture than among those who do culture?

DR. COCHI: The physicians who stated that they did not culture did not have to complete the remainder of the questionnaire, so the data on the use of antibiotics and all issues after that related to only those physicians who use throat cultures.

DR. HOUSER: If you don't have that other information, I think you should not say that culturing may increase use of antibiotics. It may actually decrease use, because all those who don't culture may treat with antibiotics.

DR. COCHI: The statements I made in that regard concerned the group of physicians who used throat cultures, which was 75% of the weighted average. It was a high percentage of the total physicians.

DR. KAPLAN: Were you able to get any data on the types of intramuscular penicillin that were used? Can you tell us how many used mixtures, how many used benzathine alone, and how many used other forms?

DR. COCHI: No, I don't have those data at this time.

DR. KAPLAN: Is it possible to get those data?

DR. COCHI : We can still get those data.

DR. SANFORD: Regarding the fact that 42% don't stop therapy when they get a negative culture, I have done similar nonrandom surveys in the treatment of urinary tract infections. I can tell you that with a negative culture fewer than 10% will stop. So the 42% figure is far better than you get with urine cultures.

DR. TOMPKINS: Once again belaboring the obvious, I would like to point out that this is merely what physicians say they do. What they actually do may be quite different. We have looked at a large number of physicians who say they culture the throat on every patient with a sore throat and found that indeed they do not always culture those patients. We have also looked at the group who say they never give penicillin unless they have a positive culture, and that's also not true. I suggest that your numbers are strikingly bad, but they are probably worse in reality.

DR. DENNY: You are speaking for internists and not pediatricians, now?

DR. TOMPKINS: Unfortunately, I always speak only for internists. But it happens to be true for pediatricians also.

DR. GERBER: Were the physicians who routinely use throat cultures asked whether they routinely reculture?

DR. COCHI: No, we didn't ask that question.

DR. HILL: Any indication how long therapy was continued?

DR. COCHI: No, we didn't ask them to specify.

DR. TOMPKINS: What are the physicians using the throat cultures for? If they start treatment without the results, and they don't stop it with the results, and they sometimes get it and sometimes don't, what is the purpose of the throat culture for those physicians?

DR. BISNO: Income enhancement.

DR. TOMPKINS: It may well be income. In a similar fashion, we had physicians look at sinus films to develop a nice logic for handling patients with potential sinusitis. When we looked at what they actually did, they never used the logic they developed. They ordered sinus films only to confirm their preconceived notion that the patient had sinusitis. They didn't change their therapy, and they didn't do anything with the patient.

I wonder if a lot of people are getting throat cultures only in those patients they are really sure have strep pharyngitis, for some intellectual confirmation of their own diagnosis rather than for a therapeutic reason.

DR. COCHI: We didn't address that issue in the survey. I think that a lot of physicians obtained a throat culture perhaps as a check on their clinical judgment or clinical skills, similar to your suggestion that it's for intellectual reasons.

DR. DAVIS: Did you assess what instruction is given to the patient? That is, does the physician contact the patient if there is a positive culture, or is it up to the patient to contact the physician? Any data there that might have something to do with continuation of antibiotics in the face of a negative culture?

DR. COCHI: We didn't get into that area at all.

DR. DILLON: I think you have raised some interesting questions about why people do things. But pediatricians have been taught to do throat cultures and that's one reason they do them. Your survey reflects this. It's reminiscent of Dr. Gordis's study some years ago that showed differences in pediatricians and family practitioners in terms of how they educated patients. This doesn't deal with the issue of whether it should or shouldn't be done, or is right or wrong. The pediatricians and the throat culture are sort of like the internist and the EKG. If you have indigestion, you better get an EKG; if you have a sore throat, you better get a throat culture. Intellectual curiosity is certainly involved, and there is also genuine concern for making as accurate a diagnosis as possible.

DR. BISNO: You could turn the data around and say that nearly 60% of physicians who take throat cultures find themselves able to discontinue antibiotics, if they had started them, when the throat culture comes back negative.

DR. SHULMAN: The survey didn't show that the 3% of physicians who *never* start antibiotics before the throat culture is positive are in this room!

DR. SCHWARTZ: I would like to bring up something that people don't write about, which I find of practical use. On one hand, academicians recommend never (or rarely) starting treatment on the day the patient is seen. The physicians in the community don't pay attention to that, with very few exceptions. I think there may be a middle ground. What I do is to buy a bottle of 1,000 penicillin pills at the beginning of the season. Each patient with high-risk criteria for group A strep gets three or four pills and starts taking them. Then, if the culture is positive, the patient is called the next day. If the culture is negative, the patient gets no other treatment. I might waste some penicillin pills, but people are loath to let children be sick that extra day, especially working parents or with school-age children.

DR. BALTIMORE: What do you accomplish by giving your patients a couple of penicillin pills?

DR. SCHWARTZ: First, my partners treat with prescription. So this gives me a face-saving way of treating. Secondly, I think that patients with group A strep improve with penicillin.

DR. MORTIMER: I have done the same thing for a long time. I think it's pretty good, partly because it may cut down transmission. On theoretic grounds, if you give benzathine penicillin on the 2d day, the patient should be culture-negative sooner.

DR. STOLLERMAN: There is something I don't think we have done well enough. Some of the data show that, by convincing people of the predictive value of a negative test, you might cut down prescriptions for an antibiotic by as much as 25%. A lot of emphasis in the literature has been that there are false-negatives, making people fear missing a positive culture.

Everybody knows that where there is a rare or low-incidence disease, negative predictive value is enormously good. In rheumatic fever, where we now have a low risk, a negative throat culture has enormous predictive value, and I don't think we have sold that very well.

A lot of people I talk to say a throat culture can be 12% wrong, based on a lot of studies of carriers, low-risk rheumatic fever areas, and so on. A negative test in a high-risk population, as in the Fort Warren studies, was 95% accurate for predictor value, if I remember right.


NEW DIAGNOSTIC PROCEDURES

DR. GERBER: How long does it take to perform the indirect ELISA test?

DR. AYOUB: Less than two hours.

DR. WASHINGTON: Two companies are working on enzyme immunoassays, Abbott and Marion. Neither sensitivity nor specificity in field trials is close to the figure you gave. We have been evaluating both and the figures are not very good at this point.

DR. HILL: What is the effect of staphylococci, which should be able to bind immunoglobulin, on the ELISA test?

DR. AYOUB: Are you referring to staphylococci like the Cowan strain that would possess Fc receptors? I don't know if anybody has looked at that.

DR. DENNY: If I were a practicing pediatrician, any

test that took an hour might as well take 24 hours. What patient will wait around in the office for an hour or two hours or three hours?

DR. MARKOWITZ: I think if you bunch them together, do a group of tests, and call the patients at the end of the day, you are much more likely to hold off therapy. Patients wouldn't have to sit around; you could telephone them.

DR. SHULMAN: As I understand it, the problem with the rapid diagnostic tests is that they are a bit too complicated for the average office practice, with centrifugations and a number of incubations.

DR. SCHWARTZ: Sometimes in winter we do 40 or 50 cultures per day in the office. Even if we took, say, 20 that were at reasonably high risk for strep, they would be spaced out throughout the morning and afternoon. To run a two-hour test, my technologist would have to begin the test at 3:00 p.m. to finish at 5:00 p.m., so it's not really an hour test because the people who come in at 9:00 a.m. still won't know the answer until 5:00 p.m. For those who come in at 9:00 a.m., I could probably pull the culture plate and give them an answer at 5:00 p.m.

DR. WASHINGTON: It's important to realize that the enzyme immunoassay is not going to be an inexpensive test. It will be even more expensive if done on an individual basis rather than in a batch. If you batch them, as with Gonazyme, you will lose a great time advantage. Dr. Denny is correct: They are rapid for the laboratory to perform on a batch process basis, but not rapid in your terms.

DR. AYOUB: The point is well taken. Indeed, it would not be cost effective on a unit basis, as with the Rotazyme. My only suggestion is that we have just started to look at these assays. They need to become much more cost effective, more readily available, and more rapid to perform.

DR. HILL: Dr. Kaplan, in regard to the C-reactive protein, you got pretty good results with 78%–80% positives in those with antibody rises, but you sort of discarded it because those who didn't have antibody rises had a relatively high rate. Weren't all your patients treated with antibiotics, and couldn't that have grossly affected the antibody responses?

DR. KAPLAN: Most of them were treated. The thing that struck us was that with a negative C-reactive protein, very few patients had a rise in antibody titer.

DR. DAJANI: Is that standard C-reactive protein or a micromethod?

DR. KAPLAN: Standard.

DR. HILL: You can do that by nephelometry now and get an answer in about 30 seconds.

DR. SCHWARTZ: There is a latex agglutination product for C-reactive protein, too, which we do in the office.

DR. HILL: I want to make a comment about the coagglutination extraction procedure for group A strep. We tried it also and were unable to show decent sensitivity.

DR. FACKLAM: Dr. Earl Edwards at the San Diego Naval Base ceased his identification of group A strep by the throat gargle and latex agglutination test because of problems with sensitivity. Pharmacia, who manufactures Phadebact reagents, still market them.

# 11

# Antibiotic Therapy: Influence of Duration, Frequency, Route of Administration, and Compliance

*Hugh C. Dillon, Jr., M.D.*

I have been asked to review antibiotic therapy for streptococcal infection from the standpoint of several important and interrelated factors that influence success in eradication of the infecting organism. These include antibiotic duration, frequency, dosage, route, and compliance. My focus will be on the rationale for and effectiveness of penicillin and alternate forms of therapy for streptococcal pharyngitis.

When we discuss streptococcal therapy, we discuss penicillin; and I will begin by reviewing the historical basis for recommended therapies. Regarding the questions posed here, recommendations were first provided by the American Heart Association (AHA) committee in 1953, around the time of penicillin's tenth birthday. Recommendations have changed relatively little over the past 30 years. It is of interest to consider how we got to where we are today and in so doing, to consider the evidence, if any, supporting the need for change.

During the war years of the 1940s, investigations were hampered by limitations in supply and by the characteristics of crystalline penicillin preparations, which required frequent injections to sustain antibacterial activity. Military requirements had priority. In civilians, penicillin was justified only in serious or life-threatening infections. Streptococcal pharyngitis clearly did not qualify, but early experience was gained in treatment of scarlet fever. Epidemic scarlet fever was a major problem during and immediately after World War II, and Table 11-1 is derived from

TABLE 11-1. Penicillin IM vs Sulfanilamide in Scarlet Fever Streptococcal Rates Before and After Rx (400 pts)

| | | Percent Pos. Gp. A Strep | | | | |
| | | Days | | | Weeks | |
| | Initial | 2 | 3 | 5 | 2 | 4 |
| --- | --- | --- | --- | --- | --- | --- |
| Penicillin IM BID 6 days | 74 | 23 | 7 | 2 | 4 | 7 |
| Penicillin IM BID 3 days | 82 | 39 | 0 | 24 | 65 | 65 |
| Sulfa P.O. 8 days | 69 | 76 | 65 | 60 | 73 | 59 |

Source: Jersild, T. 1948. Lancet 1:671.

Jersild's studies in Copenhagen between 1945–47 [1]. Twice-daily doses of 150,000 U crystalline penicillin given for six days proved remarkably effective in eradicating streptococci and in preventing recurrence. Penicillin for only three days was little more effective than sulfanilamide in preventing recurrence. Table 11–2 summarizes the conclusions of the Danish experience in over 2,000 patients. Clinical efficacy was impressive; suppurative complications, notably otitis media and mastoiditis, were eliminated and non-suppurative complications "appeared to be prevented." Dr. Jersild commented: "The length of treatment is directly related to results obtained with penicillin in scarlet fever." Others in this country and Canada subsequently confirmed the efficacy of six-day penicillin treatment in scarlet fever.

Table 11–3 depicts three separate penicillin regimens examined at Warren AFB, using procaine penicillin-in-oil at the doses and intervals shown. Men given the three-dose schedule fared best. As Stollerman's data illustrated, a 600,000 U dose of this preparation provided antistrepto-coccal activity for four to five days. The three-dose schedule in Group 1, with a 600,000 U dose on day 4, likely provided at least ten days' streptococcal therapy. Table 11–4 shows further analysis of this treatment schedule, depicting efficacy in relation to M-typeable

TABLE 11-2.  Penicillin Treatment of Scarlet Fever: Copenhagen 1945-47

Therapy with:
Crystalline penicillin 150,000 u IM six days
1.  Shortened febrile period 2-3 days
2.  Reduced recurrence rate
3.  Eliminated suppurative complications
4.  Shortened hospital stay to 8 days
5.  Appeared to prevent non-suppurative complications in 2,000 patients

Source: Jersild, T.  1948.  Lancet 1:671.

TABLE 11-3.  Streptococcal Pharyngitis--Warren AFB 1949-50: Procaine Penicillin in oil with 2% Al Mono

| Group | Unit Dose at Interval | | | | Post-Treatment Percent Gp A Strep | |
| | Stat | 48 H | 72 H | 96 H | Treated | Control |
|---|---|---|---|---|---|---|
| I | $3 \times 10^5$ | $3 \times 10^5$ | -- | $6 \times 10^5$ | 13 | 52 |
| II | $3 \times 10^5$ | -- | $3 \times 10^5$ | -- | 18 | 44 |
| III | $6 \times 10^5$ | -- | -- | -- | 31 | 57 |

Source: Denny, F. W. et al.  1950.  JAMA 143:151;
Wannamaker, L. W. et al.  1951.  Am J Med 10:673.

strains.    Treatment    eradicated    the    original    infecting serotype, which proved to be the critical factor for preventing ARF, with a cure rate of 93%.  Later acquisition of a different serotype occurred with similar frequency in treated and control groups.  Subsequent studies at Warren AFB, after benzathine penicillin G, had an even higher streptococcal eradication rate [5].

It proved more difficult to demonstrate clinical efficacy in studies of streptococcal pharyngitis than in earlier studies of more severe streptococcal infection, including scarlet    fever.    In    the    Warren    AFB    studies,    treatment

TABLE 11-4.  Streptococcal Pharyngitis--Warren AFB 1949-50: Results in Patients with M-Typeable Group A Strep Given Three Dose Schedule*

| Group I | Streptococcal Recovery Rates 3-5 Weeks Percent Positive | | |
| --- | --- | --- | --- |
| | Same Type | Diff. Type | Total |
| Treated (426 pts.) | 6.8 | 4.5 | 11.3 |
| Control (422 pts.) | 34.6 | 6.6 | 41.2 |

*Provided 9-10 days therapy
Source: Wannamaker, L. W.  1951.  Am J Med 10:673.

during the first 24 hours of illness with either penicillin or tetracycline significantly reduced fever, decreased earache, and caused a rapid return of the sedimentation rate to normal, according to studies reported by Brink and by Houser [6].  Unlike penicillin, however, tetracycline did not effectively eradicate streptococci or prevent their recurrence.  Once it was shown that the prevention of ARF was directly related to streptococcal eradication by penicillin, this became the requirement for acceptable treatment of streptococcal pharyngitis and provided the basis for the AHA recommendations some 30 years ago [7].  The criterion of streptococcal eradication with penicillin thus became the standard against which all future therapeutic regimens were measured.

Many investigators have contributed knowledge that provided a rational basis for streptococcal treatment, but we are especially indebted to Dr. Burtis Breese and his associates, notably Dr. Frank Disney, for their detailed studies in children over three decades.  Dr. Breese has retired, but Dr. Disney remains active.  Table 11-5 lists selected Breese publications, beginning in 1953, in which penicillin regimens were critically examined [8-15].  These included efficacy studies with benzathine penicillin G (BPG), comparisons of oral and intramuscular regimens, and dose-frequency studies of penicillin for streptococcal pharyngitis.

TABLE 11-5. Studies from B. B. Breese and Associates, Rochester, New York: Penicillin for Streptococcal Illness in Children

| Year Reported | Preparations and Comparisons |
|---|---|
| 1. 1953, NEJM | Benzathine Pen G I.M.--Efficacy |
| 2. 1955, Peds | Benzathine Pen G I.M.--1175 pts. |
| 3. 1956, AJDC | Phenoxymethyl Penicillin (V) efficacy |
| 4. 1957, J. Peds | Pen G Oral vs Benz. Pen G I.M. |
| 5. 1958, NEJM | Five Oral Regimens (G, V) vs BPG I.M. |
| 6. 1960, AJDC | BPG I.M.--Different preparations |
| 7. 1964, AJDC | Pen G Oral vs Synthetic Penicillin |
| 8. 1965, AJDC | Sequel to Study #5: Oral Pen G vs Benz Pen G I.M. 1180 patients |

As shown in Table 11-6 Breese and associates used specific definitions for cure, recurrence, and carriage in describing their results; and they followed acute pharyngitis patients carefully over a two-month period. Table 11-7 depicts Dr. Breese's results of a two-and-one-half year experience with a single injection of 600,000 U benzathine penicillin G in over 1,000 children, of whom 86% were considered cured [8]. An additional 8% had recurrence or became a carrier with a different serotype [9]. The corrected "cure rate" of 94% for the original infection is nearly identical to the earlier results from the Warren AFB studies. Breese commented that they were especially watchful for acute rheumatic fever and acute glomerulonephritis, but neither occurred in their patients. Pain at the injection site was the primary problem with benzathine penicillin G.

TABLE 11-6. B. B. Breese and Associates, Rochester, New York: Streptococcal Pharyngitis Studies Evaluation Methods and Definitions

| | |
|---|---|
| Cure: | Clinically well after treatment. Negative throat culture 30-61 days. |
| Recurrence: | Clinical respiratory illness plus Positive throat culture within 61 days. |
| Carrier: | Asymptomatic after treatment; throat culture positive within 61 days. |

Source: Breese, B. B., and F. A. Disney. 1955. Peds 15:516.

TABLE 11-7.  Benzathine Penicillin G I.M. Breese, 1955, Evaluated 1021
Children--1952-54

| Results | No. Patients | Percent Total |
|---|---|---|
| Cure: | 875 | 86 |
| Recurrence or carrier Different type: | 85 | 8 |
| Total cure, original infection: | 960 | 94 |
| Recurrence or carrier Same type: | 61 | 6 |

Cure vs failure rate: 94% vs. 6%

Source: Breese, B. B., and F. A. Disney.  1955.  Peds 15:516

    Breese next reported the first extensive comparison of a
600,000 U dose of benzathine penicillin G to oral penicillin G
in 483 children randomly treated with one of several regimens [11].   Oral dosage schedules were 200,000 U tablets
three times daily for either eight- or ten-days, and 200,000
U penicillin G tablets four times daily for ten days. There
was little difference between eight and ten day schedules of
thrice-daily penicillin G.   However, benzathine penicillin G
was superior to all oral regimens except the ten-day course
of oral penicillin given four times daily, for which cure
rates were identical (81%).   These reported cure rates were
not adjusted after correction for serotype differences, but
Breese reported that 40% of all bacteriologic relapses within
two months were due to a different M-type.
    In yet another careful and well-designed study [12],
these clinicians compared oral penicillin G and IM benzathine
penicillin G, to determine whether the dose and frequency
of administration of oral penicillin recommended by the AHA
committee could be altered without jeopardizing efficacy.
Table 11-8 depicts the data for the five randomly compared
treatment schedules, with the dose in units and the
frequency of dosing shown across the top.   The percentage
of cure after one month was similar for all oral regimens
(83%–89%); there was a small but significant difference in
favor of IM benzathine penicillin G (95%) over oral

TABLE 11-8. Penicillin G Oral--Four Schedules vs Benz Pen. G

| Unit dose | 200,000 | 400,000 | 400,000 | 800,000 | 600,000 |
|---|---|---|---|---|---|
| Schedule | QID | BID | QID | BID | BPG-IM |
| No. patients | 92 | 95 | 95 | 98 | 97 |
| Percent cure one month | 89 | 83 | 84 | 85 | 95* |

*BPG cure rate sig, greater, p = 0.05
Source: Breese, B. B. et al. 1965. AJDC 110:125

regimens. Further analysis showed that the clinical recurrence rate was also lowest (1%) in patients given benzathine penicillin G. These studies also provided evidence that twice-daily oral doses of 400,000 units of penicillin G compared favorably with other oral penicillin schedules using larger (up to 800,000 units) or more frequent (up to four times/day) doses. In addition, the investigators found that single dose oral therapy in 50 patients given penicillin G 800,000 U/day/10 days, yielded a failure rate of over 40%, proving this schedule to be unacceptable.

Breese again emphasized that recurrences beyond one month, whether or not symptomatic, were often due to new streptococcal serotypes and were not treatment failures per se. He stated some 20 years ago that: "Unquestionably, the most disturbing factor in the treatment of children with beta-hemolytic strep infection is the extremely high rate of recurrent episodes of clinical disease or the carriage state in children who have been treated by what are considered adequate methods" [14].

Undoubtedly, these studies were influential in leading to the increasing acceptance of oral therapy for streptococcal pharyngitis, since eradication rates had been shown to be quite similar with oral and IM benzathine penicillin G. The trend towards oral therapy was further enhanced by introduction of penicillin suspensions, conveniently packaged for ten-day dosing. Yet another factor was the very real problem of the pain on injection associated with IM benzathine penicillin G. These factors, plus the low incidence of ARF in patients given any form of penicillin treatment, were quite important in establishing therapeutic routines.

Bass and associates critically examined intramuscular penicillin therapy in studies reported in 1976, shown in Table 11-9 [16]. They compared four intramuscular penicillin regimens, using benzathine penicillin G with and without procaine penicillin. The table also includes earlier data from a similar study by Breese. With the combinations and doses shown in Table 11-9, Bass found that the 900,000 U benzathine penicillin G + 300,000 U procaine penicillin regimen was superior (94% cure rate at six weeks) to the others (79%-91%) and felt that this provided optimal therapy for children with streptococcal pharyngitis. Procaine penicillin also appeared to reduce local reactions and pain at the injection site. Breese's data, from a study done 16 years earlier, employed regimens identical to two of Bass's and was done to evaluate methods for reducing the local reactions and pain associated with benzathine penicillin G. Both he and Krugman found the addition of prednisolone to be helpful, without reducing efficacy. Both this recommendation and the use of the benzathine penicillin G-procaine mixture deserve more attention than they have received.

TABLE 11-9. Benzathine Penicillin and Benzathine plus Procaine Penicillin

| Breese et al. | No. Pts. | Percent Cure--6 weeks |
|---|---|---|
| BPG $6 \times 10^5$ | 99 | 77 |
| { BPG $6 \times 10^5$ <br> Proc. P. $6 \times 10^5$ | 108 | 72 |
| Bass et al. | | |
| BPG $6 \times 10^5$ | 100 | 79* |
| BPG $12 \times 10^5$ | 100 | 91 |
| { BPG $6 \times 10^5$ <br> Proc. P. $6 \times 10^5$ | 100 | 85 |
| { BPG $9 \times 10^5$ <br> Proc. P. $3 \times 10^5$ | 100 | 94 |

*Sig. diff. treatment failure rate, p < 0.025
Source: Breese et al. 1960. AJDC; Bass et al. 1976. JAMA.

Following the introduction of phenoxymethyl penicillin (penicillin V) in the 1950s, efficacy was quickly established in a number of studies [10], including those of Dr. Max Stillerman, also a careful clinical student of streptococcal disease in children. As shown in Table 11–10, when Dr. Stillerman compared 125 and 250 mg doses of penicillin V, he found the higher dose to be more effective in eradicating streptococci (89% vs 77%, $p < 0.001$) [17]. Of particular interest were his observations that failure or relapse rates were higher with M-typeable strains than with non-typeable strains, and that the larger dose of penicillin V was significantly more effective in their eradication ($p < 0.02$). He specifically found the highest relapse rates in infections by M-types 3, 4, 5, 6, and 12.

TABLE 11-10. Phenoxymethyl Penicillin in Streptococcal Pharyngitis Typeable and Non-Typeable Strains

| Ten-day Therapy | No. Pts. | Percent Cure One Month | |
|---|---|---|---|
| TID | | | |
| Penicillin V 125 | | | |
| M-Typeable | 121 | 72 | |
| Non-Typeable | 113 | 82 | |
| Total | 234 | 77 | |
| Penicillin V 250 | | | Sig. Diff. |
| M-Typeable | 122 | 84 | p < 0.02 |
| Non-Typeable | 86 | 95 | p < 0.001 |
| Total | 208 | 89 | p < 0.001 |

Highest relapse rate: M types 3, 4, 5, 6, 12.
Source: Stillerman, M. 1964. AJDC 107:35.

Another interesting study using penicillin V, the results of which are shown in Table 11–11, was reported by Rosenstein, Markowitz et al. [18]. Several parameters of streptococcal therapy were examined, and in addition, compliance was studied carefully by testing for penicillinuria as advocated by Gordis and Markowitz [19] in patients receiving rheumatic fever prophylaxis. In this investigation,

TABLE 11-11.  Phenoxymethyl Penicillin vs Nafcillin: Efficacy, Compliance, and Factors in Treatment Failure

| Treatment | No. Pis. | Percent Cure | Percent Positive Pen Urine Test |
|---|---|---|---|
| 400,000 U BID | | | (279/331 tested) |
| Pen V | 170 | 90 | 91 |
| Nafcillin | 161 | 86 | 84 |

Relapse rate: 15% m+; 8% m- (p = 0.01)
Highest with M-12, M-3 (p < 0.01)
Source: Rosenstein, B. J., M. Markowitz et al. 1968. Peds 73:513.

the efficacy of twice-daily oral penicillin V was confirmed, and it was further demonstrated that penicillinase-resistant penicillins such as nafcillin offered no advantages over penicillin V. Excellent compliance was documented for both drugs, and twice-daily therapy was suggested to enhance compliance. These workers, like Stillerman, observed a higher relapse rate with M-positive strains, notably types 3 and 12. While our own data have not yet been carefully analyzed, we have observed over the past three years in Birmingham a resurgence of scarlet fever, associated with an increased number of M-type 3 infection. Clinical recurrence has been more common following penicillin therapy than was the case in our earlier studies, and several instances of recurrent scarlet fever have been seen.

Because of penicillin allergy, a need for alternative therapy has been recognized. Several antibiotic agents have been compared to penicillin in treatment of strep pharyngitis, but erythromycin remains the suggested alternate for patients allergic to penicillin [20]. Erythromycin resistance is not a significant problem in this country; group A strains are susceptible with MICs of 0.005 to 0.5 mcg/ml. Table 11-12 depicts the results of Haight's early study in naval recruits with scarlet fever (type 19) at Great Lakes Naval Station in 1953 [21]. Patients received either intramuscular procaine penicillin twice daily or 200 mg erythromycin orally in six doses per day for ten days.

TABLE 11-12.  Erthromycin vs Procaine Penicillin in Scarlet Fever.
Navy Recruits--Great Lakes, 1953

| Treatment | No. Pts. | Positive Group A Strep (percent) Day | | |
|---|---|---|---|---|
| | | 2 | 10 | 16 |
| Pro Pen Ten days | 78 | 5 | 1 | 6 |
| Erythromycin 1.2 Gm Daily ten days | 78 | 5 | 1 | 5 |
| Placebo Ten days | 52 | 75 | 70 | * |

*Placebo group given treatment on day 10
Source: Haight, T. H.  1954.  J Lab Clin Med 43:15.

A placebo-treated group of 52 was added after the study began; these men received the penicillin regimen after day 10.  Streptococcal eradication rates were the same in the penicillin and erythromycin groups.  Clinical improvement was rapid in both treatment groups, with fever gone after three days; this compared to six days for fever to disappear in placebo patients.  One aim of this study was to compare immune responses; ASO rises occurred in only 14% and 10% respectively of erythromycin- and penicillin-treated groups, compared to 60% of placebo patients.  Haight concluded that neither drug permitted development of immunity, but type-specific antibody was not measured.

Data from some early studies in children comparing erythromycin and penicillin therapy are shown in Table 11-13 [22-26].  Improved efficacy with erythromycin noted in studies after 1961 was attributed to improved formulation, resulting in better absorption and higher levels.  The last three studies in the table [24-26] showed erythromycin estolate to compare favorably with oral penicillin, but with both drugs failure rates were in the range of 20%.  Moffett used two dose ranges of erythromycin, 20 mg/kg and 40 mg/kg, and found the higher dose superior [24].

TABLE 11-13. Erythromycin vs Penicillin in Children. Early Experiences

| | Percent Cure--One Month | |
| | Erthromycin | Penicillin |
|---|---|---|
| Stillerman, 1960 | 48 | 82 |
| Breese, 1961 | 64 | 73 |
| Stillerman, 1963 | 78 | 72 |
| Moffett, 1963 | 78* | 77 |
| Breese, 1966 | 85 | 80 |

*Doubled dose, efficacy = 87%

These studies were followed by a larger number, all using erythromycin estolate, reported in the 1970s and shown in Table 11–14 [27–32]; several were comparisons with penicillin. Cure rates at one month are shown in Table 11–14. As indicated, several different dosage schedules were used with similar results for each regimen and study population. In the studies comparing penicillin and erythromycin,

TABLE 11-14. Erthromycin Estolate in Streptococcal Pharyngitis: Dose, Frequency, Efficacy*

| Investigators | No. Pts. | Daily Dose (mg/kg) | Schedule | Percent Cure One month |
|---|---|---|---|---|
| 1. Howie, 1972 | 50 | (25) | TID | 92 |
| 2. Levine, 1972 | 52 | (30) | TID | 85 |
| 3. Shapera, 1973 | 34 | (40) | QID | 91 |
| | 52 | (40) | BID | 94 |
| 4. Breese, 1974 | 100 | (30) | TID | 92 |
| | 103 | (30) | BID | 85 |
| 5. Derrick, Dillon, 1976 | 97 | (20) | BID | 86 |
| 6. Breese, 1977 | 60 | (30) | TID | 83 |

*Most were comparisons with oral penicillin; no sig. diff. between drugs or schedules

streptococcal eradication rates did not differ significantly. Careful attention was paid to compliance in these studies; for example, Shapera tested antibacterial activity in urine and found such activity in 70% of orally treated patients on day 6, 7, or 8 [29].

In our study [31], a daily dose of 20mg/kg given BID was employed and compliance judged by interview during and after treatment and by measurement of residual medication after treatment. Based on these criteria, streptococcal eradication rates were 89% in 75 patients with 90% compliance, 76% in 17 patients with 75% compliance, and only 60% in five patients with 50% compliance. We also concluded that twice-daily dosing enhanced compliance.

The final erythromycin data (Table 11–15) compare results obtained with various erythromycin formulations from three studies [33–35]. Erythromycin estolate and erythromycin ethyl succinate (EES) are the preparations commonly used in children. Pharmacokinetic studies show more uniform absorption and higher blood levels in both fasting and nonfasting states with the estolate. Ryan's study from Australia indicated the estolate to be superior to the stearate, when both were given in the fasting state [33]. In Janicki's multicenter study, formulations were prescribed according to manufacturer's recommended dose, the highest dose being for EES [34]. Comparable results were obtained. Derrick and I found equivalent results when comparing recommended doses and concluded that, in prescribing erythromycin, the calculated dose should be based upon the preparation chosen [35].

Interest in the oral cephalosporins as alternative forms of therapy has been expressed. Table 11–16 summarizes data from several investigations in which cephalexin was compared to penicillin V; two studies, Matsen's [36] and ours [37], also included benzathine penicillin G. These studies, all conducted in the early 1970s, showed results with cephalexin comparable to those obtained with penicillin [36–39]. No specific advantage to using an antibiotic more expensive than penicillin was apparent. More recently, Dr. Stillerman reported in abstract form a compilation of several studies from his practice that suggested that oral cephalosporins were superior to penicillin V: 89% of 263 patients treated with a cephalosporin were cured compared to 77% of 230 patients given penicillin V, a difference significant at the 0.001 level [40]. This comparison, however, lacked the validity of a double-blind or randomized study done within a single timeframe. Currently, a collaborative double-blind study comparing penicillin and cephalexin is in progress.

TABLE 11-15. Comparison of Erythromycin Formulations: Streptococcal Pharyngitis

| | Percent Cure at One Month (dose given in mg/kg) | | |
| --- | --- | --- | --- |
| | E. Stearate | E. Estolate | EES |
| Ryan, 1973 | 84 (30-50) | 96* (30-50) | -- |
| Janicki, 1975 | 91 (30) | 96 (30) | 92 (50) |
| Derrick and Dillon, 1979 | -- | 87 (20) | 86 (40) |

*Diff. sig., p < 0.05

TABLE 11-16. Oral Cephalosporin* in Streptococcal Pharyngitis: Summary--Comparative Studies

| | | Percent Bacteriologic Cure | | |
| --- | --- | --- | --- | --- |
| Investigators | Total Pts. | Cephalosporin | P.O. Pen | BPG I.M. |
| 1. Disney, Breese, 1971 | 165 | 81 | 76 | -- |
| 2. Stillerman, M., 1970 | 75 | 91 | 86 | -- |
| 3. Gau, 1972 | 75 | 96 | 92 | -- |
| 4. Rabinovitch, 1973 | 98 | 100 | 94 | -- |
| 5. Matsen, 1974 | 122 | 97 | 97 | 96 |
| 6. Derrick, Dillon, 1974 | 227 | 96 | 92 | 95 |

*Cephalexin

In addition to Dr. Stillerman, others have noted a change in their experiences with penicillin. Schwartz and colleagues in Washington [41] recently reported their comparison of seven- and ten-day courses of penicillin V in a study in which one goal was to revalidate the AHA recommendation that ten days' treatment for streptococcal infection is required. As indicated in Table 11–17, they revalidated that recommendation. In a very well-done study, which included monitoring compliance by several methods, a ten-day course was significantly better than a seven-day course in effecting bacteriologic cure, and failure could not be attributed to poor compliance. Although the investigators felt that the 18% bacteriologic failure rate in the ten-day group was well within the range reported previously by others, they believe that it represented a change in their own practice. Over a ten-year period ending in 1978, they had recorded failure rates of around 10%. Furthermore, their clinical recurrence rate of 12% in the current report was three-fold higher than their earlier experiences. This adds to evidence accumulating from several sources, including Dr. Frank Disney, that penicillin therapy for streptococcal pharyngitis may be less satisfactory than in former years; conclusive data on this point are not yet available.

TABLE 11-17. Bacteriologic Response to Therapy Penicillin V

|  | Seven-Day Treatment Group (Percent) (N=96) | Ten-day Treatment Group (Percent) (N=95) |
|---|---|---|
| Cure | 66(69) | 78(82) |
| Failure | 30(31) | 17(18)* |
|   Relapse | 28 | 14 |
|   Indeterminate | 2 | 3 |

*p = .05

I must address specifically the issue of compliance. Patients and parents do tend to forget to take or to give medicine, or they discontinue it too soon, especially as symptoms subside. My own experience is that compliance with oral regimens for streptococcal therapy—whether for skin or throat infections—has been best in clinical investigations where patients are carefully advised and instructed, and where there is one particular nurse or physician with whom the patient can identify. This is why we attempt to have all our clinic patients being treated for streptococcal infection come to a "Streptococcal Clinic," staffed by the same nurse who coordinates streptococcal clinical investigation. Thus, all patients get the benefit of education and attention for a specific problem. Others have demonstrated that, when the disease being treated is considered significant by the patient or parent, compliance is more likely [42]. Physicians who educate patients are therefore more likely to have compliant patients. Education is a key word, and as Dr. Gordis demonstrated some years ago, physicians must be educated too. Gordis found patients of family practitioners less likely to be compliant than those cared for by pediatricians [42]. Perhaps those of us interested in streptococcal disease have done a poor job of communicating with family practitioners.

Two other points regarding optimal therapy bear mention. First, in prescribing oral suspensions, one should provide accurate dispensers to assure proper dosing. This in itself may enhance compliance. Second, twice-daily regimens are effective and perhaps should be employed more often, especially in school children and children of working mothers.

Perhaps streptococcal infection is undergoing a change in its natural history, but we must remember that antibiotic therapy has been part of this "natural history" now for over 40 years. We see less acute rheumatic fever and we also see far fewer suppurative complications—despite "bacteriologic" failures. Furthermore, "failure rates" of 20% were not uncommon in past years, especially with oral therapy, but even with benzathine penicillin G in some studies.

Thus, penicillin remains the drug of choice at this time.

REFERENCES

1. Jersild, T. 1978. Penicillin therapy in scarlet fever and complicating otitis. *Lancet* 1:671.

2. Stollerman, G.H. 1954. The use of antibiotics for the prevention of rheumatic fever. *Am J Med* 17:757.

3. Denny, F. W., L. W. Wannamaker, W. R. Brink et al. 1950. Prevention of rheumatic fever: treatment of the preceding streptococcic infection. *JAMA* 143:151.

4. Wannamaker, L. W., C. H. Rammelkamp, Jr., F. W. Denny et al. 1956. Prophylaxis of acute rheumatic fever by treatment of the preceding streptococcal infection with various amounts of depot penicillin. *Am J Med* 10:673.

5. Chamovitz, R., F. J. Catanzaro, C. A. Stetson et al. 1954. Prevention of rheumatic fever by treatment of previous streptococcal infections: I. Evaluation of benza-

thine penicillin G. *New Engl J Med* 251:466.

6. Brink, W. R., C. H. Rammelkamp, Jr., F. W. Denny et al. 1951. Effect of penicillin and aureomycin on the natural course of streptococcal tonsillitis and pharyngitis. *Am J Med* 10:300.

7. Jones, T. D. 1955. Chairman, Committee on Prevention of Rheumatic Fever and Bacterial Endocarditis of the American Heart Association: Prevention of Rheumatic Fever and Bacterial Endocarditis Through Control of Streptococcal Infections. *Circulation* 11:317.

8. Breese, B. B. 1953. Treatment of beta hemolytic streptococcic infections in the home. *JAMA* 152:10.

9. Breese, B. B., and F. A. Disney. 1955. The successful treatment of beta hemolytic streptococcal infections in children with a single injection of repository penicillin (benzathine penicillin G). *Pediatrics* 15:516.

10. Breese, B. B., and F. A. Disney. 1956. Penicillin V treatment of beta hemolytic streptococcal infections in children. *Am J Dis Child* 92:20.

11. Breese, B. B., and F. A. Disney. 1957. A comparison of intramuscular and oral benzathine penicillin G in the treatment of streptococcal infections in children. *J Pediatr* 51:157.

12. Breese, B. B., and F. A. Disney. 1958. Penicillin in the treatment of streptococcal infections: a comparison of five different oral and one parenteral form. *New Engl J Med* 259:57.

13. Breese, B. B., F. A. Disney, and W. B. Talpey. 1960. Improvement in local tolerance and therapeutic effectiveness of benzathine penicillin. *Am J Dis Child* 99:149.

14. Breese, B. B., F. A. Disney, and W. B. Talpey. 1964. Beta hemolytic streptococcal infections in children. *Am J Dis Child* 107:232.

15. Breese, B. B., F. A. Disney, and W. B. Talpey. 1965. Penicillin in streptococcal infections. *Am J Dis Child* 110:125.

16. Bass, J. W., F. W. Crast, C. P. Knowles et al. 1976. Streptococcal pharyngitis in children: a comparison of four treatment schedules with intramuscular penicillin G benzathine. *JAMA* 235:1112.

17. Stillerman, M., S. H. Bernstein. 1964. Streptococcal pharyngitis therapy. *Am J Dis Child* 107:35.

18. Rosenstein, B. J., M. Markowitz, E. Goldstein et al. 1968. Factors involved in treatment failures following oral penicillin therapy of streptococcal pharyngitis. *J Pediatr* 73:513.

19. Markowitz, M., and L. Gordis. 1968. A mail-in

technique for detecting penicillin inurine. *Pediatrics* 41:151.

20. Kaplan, E. L. 1977. Chairman, American Heart Association Committee on Rheumatic Fever and Bacterial Endocarditis: Prevention of Rheumatic Fever. *Circulation* 55:S1–4.

21. Haight, T. H. 1954. Erythromycin therapy of respiratory infections: I. Controlled studies on the comparative efficacy of erythromycin and penicillin in scarlet fever. *J Lab Clin Med* 43:15.

22. Stillerman, M., S. H. Bernstein, M. L. Smith et al. 1960. Antibiotics in the treatment of beta hemolytic streptococcal pharyngitis: factors influencing the results. *Pediatrics* 25:27.

23. Stillerman, M., S. H. Bernstein, M. Smith et al. 1963. Erythromycin propionate and potassium penicillin V in the treatment of group A streptococcal pharyngitis. *Pediatrics* 31:22.

24. Moffett, H. L., H. G. Cramblett, J. P. Black et al. 1963. Erythromycin estolate and phenoxymethyl penicillin in the treatment of streptococcal pharyngitis. *Antimicrob Agents Chemother* 3:759.

25. Breese, B. B., F. A. Disney, and W. B. Talpey. 1961. Triacetyloleandomycin—a substitute for penicillin G. *Am J Dis Child* 101:423.

26. Breese, B. B., F. A. Disney, and W. B. Talpey. 1966. Beta-hemolytic streptococcal illness: a comparison of the effectiveness of penicillin G, triacetyloleandomycin and erythromycin estolate. *Am J Dis Child* 111:128.

27. Howie, V. M., and J. H. Ploussard. 1976. Compliance dose-response relationships on streptococcal pharyngitis. *Am J Dis Child* 123:18.

28. Levine, M. K., and J. D. Berman. A comparison of clindamycin and erythromycin in beta-hemolytic streptococcal infections. *J Med Assoc Ga* 61:108.

29. Shapera, R. M., K. A. Hable, and J. M. Matsen. 1973. Erythromycin therapy twice daily for streptococcal pharyngitis. *JAMA* 226:531.

30. Breese, B. B., F. A. Disney, W. B. Talpey et al. 1974. Streptococcal infections in children: comparison of the therapeutic effectiveness of erythromycin administered twice-daily with erythromycin, penicillin phenoxymethyl and clindamycin administered three times daily. *Am J Dis Child* 128:457.

31. Derrick, C. W., and H. C. Dillon. 1976. Erythromycin therapy for streptococcal pharyngitis. *Am J Dis Child* 130:175.

32. Breese, B. B., F. A. Disney, J. L. Green et al.

1977. The treatment of beta hemolytic streptococcal pharyngitis: comparison of amoxicillin, erythromycin estolate and penicillin V. *Clin Pediatr (Phila.)* 16:460.

33. Ryan, D., G. H. Dreher, and J. A. Hurst. 1973. Estolate and stearate forms of erythromycin in the treatment of acute beta hemolytic streptococcal pharyngitis. *Med J Aust* 1:20.

34. Janicki, R. S., J. C. Garnham, M. C. Worland et al. 1975. Comparison of erythromycin ethylsuccinate, stearate and estolate treatments of group A streptococcal infections of the upper respiratory tract. *Clin Pediatr (Phila.)* 14:1098.

35. Derrick, C. W., and H. C. Dillon. 1979. Streptococcal pharyngitis therapy: a comparison of two erythromycin formulations. *Am J Dis Child* 133:1146.

36. Matsen, J. M., O. Torstenson, S. E. Siegel et al. 1974. Use of available dosage forms of cephalexin in clinical comparison with phenoxymethyl penicillin and benzathine penicillin in the treatment of streptococcal pharyngitis in children. *Antimicrob Agents Chemother* 6:501.

37. Derrick, C. W., and H. C. Dillon. 1974. Therapy for prevention of acute rheumatic fever. *Circulation* 50(3):38.

38. Disney, F. A., B. B. Breese, J. L. Green et al. 1971. Cephalexin and penicillin therapy of childhood beta-hemolytic streptococcal infections. *Postgrad Med J* 47 (February):47.

39. Stillerman, M., and H. D. Isenberg. 1970. Streptococcal pharyngitis therapy: comparison of cyclacillin, cephalexin and potassium penicillin V. *Antimicrob Agents Chemother* 10:270.

40. Stillerman, M. 1979. Comparison of cefaclor and penicillin V potassium in group A streptococcal pharyngitis. Interscience Conference on Antimicrobial Agents and Chemotherapy. Abstract 529.

41. Schwartz, R. H., R. L. Wientzen, F. Pedreria et al. 1981. Penicillin V for group A streptococcal pharyngotonsillitis. *JAMA* 246:1790.

42. Gordis, L., M. Markowitz, and A. M. Lilienfeld. 1969. Why patients don't follow medical advice: a study of children on long-term antistreptococcal prophylaxis. *J Pediatr* 75:957.

# 12

# Management of Streptococcal Pharyngitis: Choice of Antibiotics with Regard to Adverse Reactions and Bacteriological Failures

*Theodore C. Eickhoff, M.D.*

The bacteriologic failures and adverse reactions encountered in the antibiotic management of streptococcal pharyngitis can best be reviewed by summarizing the data in the literature for specific drugs that have been extensively studied in clinical trials. I will review first the several penicillins that have been used, including benzathine penicillin G, penicillin V, ampicillin, and amoxycillin. This will be followed by the cephalosporins, cephalexin, and cephradine. The erythromycins and clindamycin will then be reviewed. Finally, I will briefly discuss some of the factors that may contribute to bacteriologic failure.

## PENICILLINS

Benzathine penicillin G is unquestionably the most generally recommended drug to treat streptococcal pharyngitis. The eradication rate of Group A beta-hemolytic streptococci from the pharynx, evaluated at 60-day follow-up, had generally been about 90%–95% [1,2], although a clinical and bacteriologic cure rate of only 72% was reported by Howie and Ploussard in 1971 [3]. Adverse reactions have generally been reported with a frequency of 1%–5%, although local pain has been reported in up to 50% of recipients of benzathine penicillin G [4]. Local pain can be sharply diminished by the use of procaine in the preparation; this has led to occasional problems with adverse reactions due to the procaine component.

The optimal dosage of benzathine penicillin G preparations was extensively studied by Bass and his colleagues in 400 children 6 months to 14 years old [5]. Their data suggested that the optimal dose of benzathine penicillin G should exceed 600,000 units, but need not exceed 1.2 million units. Indeed, optimal results were obtained with a combination of 900,000 units of benzathine penicillin G and 300,000 units of procaine penicillin.

Penicillin G, given orally, has also proven satisfactory in treatment, as long as the dose was sufficient. Eradication rates of 85%–90% have been reported [2,6,7]; although satisfactory, these rates have generally been slightly less than those achieved by adequate dosage of benzathine penicillin G.

Oral penicillin V, from 500 to 1000 mg/day, has similarly proved satisfactory [7–11]. Eradication rates have ranged from 80%–90%, comparable to those reported for penicillin G. In a recent study, Schwartz et al. [12] reported that seven days of penicillin V therapy resulted in a 31% failure rate, whereas the recommended ten full days of therapy was associated with a failure rate of only 18%.

Other studies of the influence of duration of therapy on bacteriologic cure rates of group A beta-hemolytic streptococcal pharyngitis generally support the validity of the recommended ten days of therapy. Less than ten days of oral therapy has resulted in eradication rates of 50% to 80%, whereas ten full days of therapy has resulted in eradication rates of 80%–90% [13,14]. Similar data were reported by Breese, using intramuscular procaine penicillin [15].

In 1972, Colcher and Bass reported what they considered to be optimal oral penicillin therapy for streptococcal pharyngitis [16]. In a group of 100 children given 250 mg penicillin V t.i.d. for ten days, the total failure and relapse rate was 25%, and only 58% of subjects had antibacterial activity in their urine on day 9. In a similar group of 100 children given the same medication schedule, and in addition counseled regarding the importance of completing a full ten-day course of the drug, the total failure and relapse rate was only 10%, and 80% of subjects had antibacterial activity in their urine on day 9.

Both ampicillin and amoxycillin have been evaluated in a number of trials. Doses used have been variable, but generally about 50 mg/kg/day for ampicillin, and 20 mg/kg/day for amoxycillin [6,8–10,17–19]. Failure rates compare with those in studies of other oral penicillins, including penicillin G and V, and generally range from 10%–25%.

## CEPHALOSPORINS

The oral cephalosporins have been evaluated far less extensively in the management of streptococcal phayrngitis than the oral penicillins, and the number of subjects reported in the literature is relatively few. Nevertheless, eight studies of cephalexin and cephradine in the management of streptococcal pharyngitis have yielded failure rates ranging from 3% to 19% [8,9–24]. Thus, one may conclude that oral cephalosporins are at least as effective as oral penicillins in the eradication of group A beta-hemolytic streptococci, although such therapy is substantially more expensive than therapy with oral penicillins

## ERYTHROMYCINS

Virtually all the erythromycin preparations have been studied in management of streptococcal pharyngitis, and all have yielded failure rates from 5%–15% [25–29]. For example, Ryan reported a 2% failure rate among subjects treated with erythromycin estolate, and a 14% failure rate in subjects concurrently treated with erythromycin stearate [25]. Shapera et al. found a 7% failure rate among 86 subjects treated with erythromycin estolate [26]. Failure rates with erythromycin ethylsuccinate have ranged from 10% reported by Hughes [27], to 6%, reported by Janicke [28]. Derrick and Dillon [29] reported recently that 20 mg/kg/day of erythromycin estolate, in a controlled trial, achieved a cure rate essentially identical to that achieved with 40 mg/kg/day erythromycin ethylsuccinate.

Eradication rates with erythromycins thus have been generally excellent, equivalent to or even exceeding those achieved with oral penicillins. The principle problem with erythromycin has been gastrointestinal intolerance reported in as many as 25% of recipients. Predictably, 5%–10% of erythromycin recipients will experience such severe gastrointestinal intolerance that they are unable to continue the drug.

## LINCOMYCIN AND CLINDAMYCIN

Lincomycin has been evaluated in the management of streptococcal pharyngitis and is effective; it has, however, been totally supplanted by clindamycin, and therefore will not be discussed further.

Clindamycin has been extensively evaluated in several hundred patients with streptococcal pharyngitis, with eradication rates in the range of 80%–95% [17,30–33]. It thus appears that clindamycin is as effective in the management of streptococcal pharyngitis as are the penicillins, the cephalosporins, and erythromycins. The frequency of adverse reactions to clindamycin reported in these and other studies [34] has varied from 0 to 30% or more, consisting, of course, primarily of gastrointestinal intolerance, diarrhea, and pseudomembranous enterocolitis. Clindamycin represents effective oral therapy of streptococcal pharyngitis, although it would seem to be indicated only rarely.

## FACTORS THAT MAY CONTRIBUTE TO BACTERIOLOGIC FAILURE OF TREATMENT

### Role of Penicillinase-Producing *Staphylococcus aureus*

The possibility that penicillinase-producing *Staphylococcus aureus*, present in the pharyngeal or tonsillar flora, interferes with the bactericidal activity of penicillin against group A beta-hemolytic streptococci was suggested in the Scandinavian literature in the late 1950s. Among the first in the United States to suggest such a phenomenon were Frank and Miller [35], who described a patient with prolonged pharyngitis associated with the continued presence in the pharynx of a M-Type 6 group A beta-hemolytic streptococcus, together with penicillinase-producing *S. aureus*. Substantial doses of oral penicillin failed to eradicate either organism, even after two weeks of therapy. When therapy was changed to erythromycin, both organisms were eradicated promptly. As a result of this experience, these investigators suggested that penicillinase-producing staphylococci present locally in the pharynx or on the tonsils might inactivate penicillinase-susceptible penicillins and thus reduce the concentration of active drug in the area to levels below those necessary to kill group A streptococci.

Kundsin and Miller [36] subsequently reported their experience in over 200 patients with streptococcal pharyngitis and supported this possibility by finding a relative excess of treatment failures among patients concurrently colonized with penicillinase-producing staphylococci, in contrast to those colonized by staphylococci not producing penicillinase.

In contrast, Quie and his colleagues [37] reviewed their data regarding approximately 140 children with streptococcal pharyngitis and found no correlation between the treatment failure rate and the presence or absence of penicillinase-producing staphylococci.

Markowitz et al. [38] approached the problem differently and compared the efficacy of nafcillin and penicillin V in children with streptococcal pharyngitis. They subsequently analyzed their data in relation to the concurrent presence or absence of pharyngeal penicillinase-producing S. *aureus*. Among children with streptococcal pharyngitis, but without pharyngeal penicillinase-producing staphylococci, penicillin V resulted in an 8% failure rate, and nafcillin in a 14% failure rate. Among children with streptococcal pharyngitis and concurrent pharyngeal penicillinase-producing staphylo-ylococci, the failure rate was 19% with penicillin V therapy and 14% with nafcillin therapy. Because of the small numbers of patients with streptococcal pharyngitis and penicillinase-producing staphylococci in the pharynx, the authors concluded that this possible difference in effectiveness of penicillin V versus nafcillin was not significant.

Thus, the precise role of pharyngeal penicillinase-producing staphylococci as a factor contributing to bacteriologic treatment failure remains in dispute. We now know, of course, that a variety of other organisms commonly present in the pharynx also produce beta-lactamases, and may account for these discrepant conclusions at least in part. Anaerobic organisms are almost invariably present on the pharyngeal surface or in tonsillar tissue, producing beta-lactamase activity. Some insight into the role of beta-lactamase activity generated by anaerobes was gained from the recent report of Brook and Leyva [39], who studied the surface tonsillar flora of 20 chronic carriers of group A beta-hemolytic streptococci, and subsequently treated them with clindamycin. A ten-day course of clindamycin eradicated group A streptococcal carriage in all 20 patients and resulted in a profound reduction in the anaerobic flora on the tonsillar surface.

Penicillinase-producing strains of *Haemophilus influenzae* are commonly found in many parts of the United States today, but the possible role of this beta-lactamase activity in the treatment of streptococcal pharyngitis has not yet been evaluated.

Tolerance

The rapid bactericidal action of penicillin against group A beta-hemolytic streptococci has rarely been questioned. Allen and Sprunt [40], however, reported in 1978 that 12 strains of group A beta-hemolytic streptococci isolated from patients had a penicillin G MIC/MBC ratio that varied from 8- to 32-fold. This finding has not been extensively pursued, but such results at least raise the question whether the phenomenon of "tolerance" is a factor that contributes to failure of eradication of group A beta-hemolytic streptococci.

## CONCLUSIONS

Intramuscular benzathine penicillin G remains the "gold standard" of therapy of streptococcal pharyngitis, resulting in eradication rates of 90% or more. We have heard evidence at this conference, however, that this "therapy of choice" is actually used by practitioners in the United States for a very small minority of patients with streptococcal pharyngitis. The frequency of anaphylactic reactions to benzathine penicillin G is of the order of 1 per 100,000 doses, a rate not dissimilar to current rates of rheumatic fever in the United States.

Results achieved with benzathine penicillin G may be approached or even equalled with several kinds of oral therapy, when coupled with strong emphasis on the necessity of completing ten full days of therapy. Both penicillin G and penicillin V are acceptable, as are ampicillin and amoxycillin; no clear indication, however, exists for the latter two drugs. Oral cephalosporins, particularly cephalexin and cephradine, are equally acceptable, but again, no clear indications would seem to exist for oral cephalosporin therapy. All of the commonly used erythromycin preparations are acceptable, and erythromycin should remain the recommended alternative drug in the event of penicillin allergy. Clindamycin is similarly acceptable, but indicated only in the unusual instance of definite allergy to both penicillins and cephalosporins, and intolerance to erythromycin.

Beta-lactamase production in the pharynx or tonsils by a variety of organisms, including staphylococci, anaerobes, and possibly *H. influenzae* may adversely effect the results of therapy with penicillinase-susceptible beta-lactam drugs, but the evidence is not wholly convincing. Finally, if eradication of chronic group A beta-hemolytic streptococcal carriage is a desirable goal, which it may not be, then additional comparative trials of erythromycin, clindamycin, and possibly the cephalosporins in chronic streptococcal carriers will be needed to establish optimal therapy.

# REFERENCES

1. Chamovitz, R., F. J. Catanzaro, C. A. Stetson et al. 1954. Prevention of rheumatic fever by treatment of previous streptococcal infections. I. Evaluation of benzathine penicillin G. *New Engl J Med* 251:465–71.

2. Breese, B. B., F. A. Disney, and W. B. Talpey. 1965. Penicillin in streptococcal infections. Total dose and frequency of administration. *Amer J Dis Child* 110 (August):125–30.

3. Howie, V. M., and J. H. Ploussard. 1971. Treatment of Group A streptococcal pharyngitis in children. Comparison of lincomycin and penicillin G given orally and benzathine penicillin G given intramuscularly. *Amer J Dis Child* 121 (June):477–80.

4. Markowitz, M. 1980. Benzathine penicillin G after thirty years. *Clinical Therapeutics* 3:49–61.

5. Bass, J. W., F. W. Crast, C. R. Knowles, and C. N. Onufer. 1976. Streptococcal pharyngitis in children. A comparison of four treatment schedules with intramuscular penicillin G benzathine. *JAMA* 235:1112–16.

6. Breese, B. B., F. A. Disney, and W. B. Talpey. 1966. Beta-hemolytic streptococcal illness. Comparison of lincomycin, ampicillin, and potassium penicillin G in treatment. *Amer J Dis Child* 112:21–27.

7. Edmond, E. W., H. G. Cramblett, C. M. F. Siewers, J. Crews, B. Ellis, and G. R. Jenkins. 1966. Comparison of efficacy of phenoxymethyl penicillin and buffered penicillin G in treatment of streptococcal pharyngitis. *Journal of Pediatrics* 68 (March):442–47.

8. Stillerman, M., H. D. Isenberg, and M. Moody. 1972. Streptococcal pharyngitis therapy. Comparison of cephalexin, phenoxymethyl penicillin, and ampicillin. *Amer J Dis Child* 123:457–61.

9. Stillerman, M., H. D. Isenberg, and R. R. Facklam. 1974. Use of Amoxicillin in various respiratory infections: pharyngitis. Treatment of pharyngitis associated with group A streptococcus: comparison of amoxicillin and potassium phenoxymethyl penicillin. *Journal of Infectious Diseases* 129:S169–77.

10. Breese, B. B., F. A. Disney, W. B. Talpey, and J. L. Green. 1974. Treatment of streptococcal pharyngitis with amoxicillin. *Journal of Infectious Diseases* 129:S178–80.

11. Spitzer, T. Q., and B. A. Harris. 1977. Penicillin V therapy for streptococcal pharyngitis: Comparison of dosage schedules. *Southern Medical Journal* 70:41–42.

12. Schwartz, R. H., R. L. Wientzen, Jr., F. Pedreira

et al. 1981. Penicillin V for group A streptococcal pharyngotonsillitis. A randomized trial of seven vs ten days' therapy. *JAMA* 246:1790–95.

13. Mohler, D. N., D. G. Wallin, E. G. Dreyfus et al. 1956. Studies in the home treatment of streptococcal disease. II. A comparison of the efficacy of oral administration of penicillin and intramuscular injection of benzathine penicillin in the treatment of streptococcal pharyngitis. *New Eng J Med* 254:45–50.

14. Green, J. L., S. P. Ray, and E. Charney. 1969. Recurrence rate of streptococcal pharyngitis related to oral penicillin. *J Pediatr* 75:292–94.

15. Breese, B. B. 1953. Treatment of beta-hemolytic streptococcic infections in the home: relative value of available methods. *JAMA* 152:10–14.

16. Colcher, I. S., and J. W. Bass. 1972. Penicillin treatment of streptococcal pharyngitis. A comparison of schedules and the role of specific counseling. *JAMA* 222:657–59.

17. Jackson, H. 1973. Prevention of rheumatic fever. A comparative study of clindamycin palmitate and ampicillin in the treatment of group A beta-hemolytic streptococcal pharyngitis. *Clinical Pediatrics* 12:501–3.

18. Breese, B. B., F. A. Disney, J. L. Green, and W. B. Talpey. 1977. The treatment of beta-hemolytic streptococcal pharyngitis. Comparison of amoxicillin, erythromycin estolate, and penicillin V. *Clinical Pediatrics* 16:460–63.

19. Caloza, D. L., and G. E. Bernfeld. 1978. Two alternatives to penicillin therapy for streptococcal tonsillopharyngitis. *Current Therapeutic Research* 24:452:57.

20. Matsen, J. M., O. Torstenson, S. E. Siegel, and H. Bacaner. 1974. Use of available dosage forms of cephalexin in clinical comparison with phenoxymethyl penicillin and benzathine penicillin in the treatment of streptococcal pharyngitis in children. *Antimicrobial Agents and Chemotherapy* 6:501–6.

21. Aximi, P. H., H. G. Gramblett, A. J. de Rosario, H. Kronfol, R. E. Haynes, and M. D. Hilty. 1972. Cephalexin: treatment of streptococcal pharyngitis. *Pediat Pharm Therapy* 80:1042–45.

22. Disney, F. A., B. B. Breese, J. L. Green, W. B. Talpey, and J. R. Tobin. 1971. Cephalexin and penicillin therapy of childhood beta-hemolytic streptococcal infections. *Postgrad Med J* 47:47–51.

23. Gau, D. W., R. F. H. Horn, R. M. Solomon, and P. Johnson. 1972. Streptococcal tonsillitis in general practice: A comparison of ephalexin and penicillin therapy.

*Practitioner* 208:276–81.

24. Leiderman, E., F. R. Stowe, and W. J. Mogabgab. 1970. Cephaloglycin and cephalexin in beta-hemolytic streptococcal pharyngitis. *Clinical Medicine* 77:27–32.

25. Ryan, D. C., G. H. Dreher, and J. A. Hurst. 1973. Estolate and stearate forms of erythromycin in the treatment of acute beta-hemolytic streptococcal pharyngitis. *Medical Journal of Australia* 1:20.

26. Shapera, R. M., K. A. Hable, and J. M. Matsen. 1973. Erythromycin therapy twice daily for streptococcal pharyngitis. *JAMA* 226:531–35.

27. Hughes, W. T., and R. N. Collier. 1969. Streptococcal pharyngitis. *Amer J Dis Child* 118:700–707.

28. Janicki, R. S., J. C. Garnham, M. C. Borland, W. E. Grundy, and J. R. Thomas. 1975. Comparison of erythromycin ethyl succinate, stearate and estolate treatments of group A streptococcal infections of the upper respiratory tract. *Clinical Pediatrics* 14:1098–1107.

29. Derrick, E. W., and H. C. Dillon. 1979. Streptococcal pharyngitis therapy. A comparison of two erythromycin formulations. *Am J Dis Child* 133:1146–48.

30. Chernack, W. J., G. Leidy, R. S. Asnes, B. Grebin, and K. Sprunt. 1976. Comparison of oral clindamycin to oral and intramuscular (benzathine) penicillin in the treatment of streptococcal pharyngitis. *Current Therapeutic Research* 19:11–19.

31. Sinanian, R., G. Ruoff, J. Panzer, and W. Atkinson. 1972. Streptococcal pharyngitis: A comparison of the eradication of the organism by 5- and 10-day antibiotic therapy. *Current Therapeutic Research* 14:716–20.

32. Levine, M. K., and J. D. Berman. 1972. A comparison of clindamycin HC[1] and erythromycin estolate in beta-hemolytic streptococcal infection. *Journal of Medical Association of Georgia* 61:108–11.

33. Stillerman, M., H. D. Isenberg, and R. R. Facklam. 1973. Streptococcal pharyngitis therapy: Comparison of clindamycin palmitate and potassium phenoxymethyl penicillin. *Antimicrobial Agents and Chemotherapy* 4: 514–20.

34. Dhawan, V. K., and H. Thadepalli. 1982. Clindamycin: A review of fifteen years of experience. *Reviews of Infectious Diseases* 4:1133–52.

35. Frank, P. F., and L. F. Miller. 1962. Antagonistic effect of a penicillinase-producing staphylococcus on penicillin therapy of a streptococcal throat infection. *American Journal of the Medical Sciences* 243:582–85.

36. Kundsin, R. B., and J. M. Miller. 1964. Significance of the staphylococcus aureus carrier state in the treatment of disease due to group A streptococci. *New*

*Engl J Med* 271:1395–97.

37. Quie, P. G., H. C. Pierce, and L. W. Wannamaker. 1966. Influence of penicillinase-producing staphylococci on the eradication of group A streptococci from the upper respiratory tract by penicillin treatment. *Pediatrics* 37: 467–76.

38. Markowitz, M., I. Kramer, E. Goldstein, A. Perlman, D. Klein, R. Kramer, M. L. Blue, G. Pelovitz, and M. Roseman. 1967. Persistence of group A streptococci as related to penicillinase-producing staphylococci: Comparison of penicillin V potassium and sodium nafcillin. *Journal of Pediatrics* 71:132–37.

39. Brook, I., and F. Leyva. 1981. The treatment of the carrier state of group A beta-hemolytic streptococci with clindamycin. *Chemotherapy* 27:360–67.

40. Allen, J. L., and K. Sprunt. 1978. Discrepancy between minimum inhibitory and minimum bactericidal concentrations of penicillin for group A and group B beta-hemolytic streptococci. *Journal of Pediatrics* 93:69–71.

# 13

# Group A Streptococcal Carriers and Contacts: (When) Is Retreatment with Antibiotics Necessary?

*Edward L. Kaplan, M.D.*

## INTRODUCTION

Among the most perplexing dilemmas associated with the group A beta-hemolytic streptococcus is that of the so-called upper respiratory tract carrier. Whether it is the clinician caring for an individual patient, the public health authority faced with a community outbreak in a school or a hospital, or the laboratory scientist searching for the still-elusive pathogenetic relationship between the group A streptococcus and its nonsuppurative sequelae (acute rheumatic fever or acute nephritis), the streptococcal carrier is a problem. To understand this problem and to manage the group A streptococcal upper respiratory tract carrier practically, four questions should be addressed: (1) How can one define the group A streptococcal carrier? (2) What is the evidence that the carrier so-defined exists? (3) If there are carriers, why are they singled out as being different? What are the clinical and epidemiological implications or consequences of the streptococcal carrier state? And finally, (4) How should the carrier be managed from a practical point of view? Is eradication of the group

The recent studies carried out in the author's laboratory were supported in part by the Dwan Family Fund and in part by a grant from the National Institutes of Health (HL 19307).

A streptococcus from the upper respiratory tract of the carrier necessary?

## WHAT IS A STREPTOCOCCAL CARRIER?

First, we must agree to a definition of the term "carrier" as it relates to the group A streptococcus. This has been one of the past stumbling blocks in discussing this issue. In the literature, the terms "harbor," "carry," and "colonize" have been used interchangably. Especially confusing as well are the numerous adjectives used to modify the term carrier: for example, healthy, transient, symptomatic, convalescent, contact, intermittent, harmless, and post-infectious, to name just a few [1]. Each has a different connotation. Hamburger, for example, used "carrier" as an all-inclusive term: "The term carrier is used to indicate anyone who harbors hemolytic streptococci in the nose or throat regardless of the presence or absence of active infection" [2]. At the other end of the spectrum are Kuttner and Krumweide who stated that "one of the most difficult problems confronting physicians interested in the control of infectious diseases is that of postinfection and healthy carriers. The epidemiology of diseases associated with streptococci is particularly baffling because of the frequent occurrence of these microorganisms in the throats of normal individuals" [3].

The possibility that important differences exist even among carriers is suggested by data collected forty years ago by Kuttner and Krumweide [3]. They discussed three types of carriers: "chronic healthy" (healthy children found incidentally to harbor streptococci on admission to their study), "post-infection" (those who continue to harbor the organism after an observed acute infection), and "contact" (those who without developing clinical or laboratory evidence of streptococcal infection acquired the organism while under observation). Although the data lack a certain precision and there must be some overlap among groups, if one looks at the duration of colonization for these three categories of carriers (Figure 13–1), the intervals required for 50% of patients to lose the organism spontaneously from the upper respiratory tract are different the groups (from one month to five months). While there are loopholes in these definitions, the data suggest a need to evaluate different types of carriers.

In an attempt to clarify this issue, we propose two definitions. *Bona fide infection* includes the presence of group A streptococci in the upper respiratory tract plus evidence of host recognition (an antibody response). In

Figure 13–1. Comparison of the duration of "colonization with hemolytic streptococci in three types of "carriers."

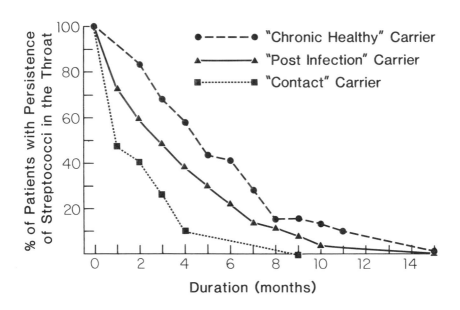

contrast, a *streptococcal carrier* is defined as one in whom group A streptococci are recovered from the upper respiratory tract, without evidence of an ongoing immune response (as measured by streptococcal antibodies). It is important that, at this point, no distinction has been made between those who have clinical signs or symptoms and those who are clinically negative. Therefore, in any population, it must be remembered that prevalence is the sum of those with infection and those who are carriers.

## DO STREPTOCOCCAL CARRIERS REALLY EXIST?

The next step is to evaluate the evidence that the streptococcal carrier as defined exists. Are there patients, asymptomatic or symptomatic, who harbor the organism but mount no host response?

One could cite a number of examples to support this concept, including data from our own laboratory [4]. Of 167 children with symptomatic pharyngitis and throat cultures positive for group A streptococci, 43% showed a rise in either antistreptolysin O or anti-DNase B titer, but

57% did not. When we added a third antibody determination (in this instance, antibody to group A carbohydrate), the percentage who failed to show an immune response dropped to 46% [5]. Therefore, approximately half of these symptomatic children with pharyngitis were infected and half were carriers. Another example of carriers with colonization of the upper respiratory tract and an absent immune response is the data published by Packer and colleagues in the late 1950s from an orphanage in Memphis [6] in which falling antistreptolysin O titers were seen in individuals who continued to harbor group A streptococci. These two studies document that carriers exist as defined here.

## WHAT ARE THE CLINICAL/EPIDEMIOLOGIC IMPLICATIONS OF THE CARRIER STATE?

Is it necessary or useful to differentiate true infection from the carrier state? In other words, what are the clinical and epidemiologic consequences of the group A streptococcal carrier state as we have defined it? Group A streptococcal infections may result in nonsuppurative sequelae. Treatment and elimination of the organism from individuals with streptococcal infection reduce the risk of attack. Does the carrier continue to pose a risk to himself (rheumatic fever) or to others (spread)? Does one reduce the risks of sequelae by treating the carrier with antibiotics?

The concept of the streptococcal carrier remains a mysterious biological phenomenon. As seen in Figure 13–2, infection occurs with rapidly multiplying organisms known to evoke a brisk host immune response and to result in nonsuppurative sequelae. For reasons that remain unclear, in some instances, the relationship between the human host and this bacterium changes dramatically. The carrier state, we propose, results in no immune response. Furthermore, it has been suggested that the risk of clinical nonsuppurative sequelae from this symbiotic relationship is substantially reduced. Whether these changes are related to human host factors or to differences in the bacterium itself remains unknown but allows interesting speculation.

For example, Mozziconacci and colleagues [7], in attempting to invoke genetics to explain the carrier state, even suggested a protective effect of individuals with blue eyes against transition to the carrier state! On the other hand, in one of the few relevant studies evaluating bacterial factors responsible for the transition, Krause and Rammelkamp [8] suggested that changes occurring in the organism during the transition to the carrier state (a temporary lack of M protein production) rendered the

Figure 13–2. Schematic representation of the transition from bona fide streptococcal pharyngitis to the streptococcal carrier state.

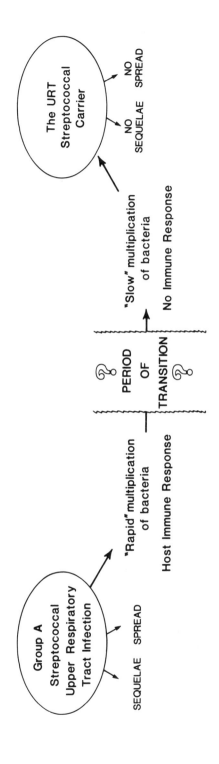

organism less infectious when inoculated into the throats of nonhuman primates.

Can it really be said that streptococcal carriers are unlikely or less likely to spread the organism to their close contacts? If true, this fact would influence the zeal with which many physicians pursue carriers.

Forty years ago Coburn and Pauli [9] indicated that this was the case, observing that "carriers of this organism usually do not communicate disease and they may usually be considered harmless. This applies to most carriers throughout the year." The studies of Kuttner and Krumweide [3] also suggested the low communicability of the carrier. The healthy asymptomatic patient seldom was responsible for spread of streptococci in their study.

However, confusion about the risk of spread posed by the carrier was fostered by the introduction of the concept of the "dangerous nasal carrier" [2] which appears to be a misnomer. Many past investigators have indicated that, in contrast to throat carriers, nasal "carriers" are frequently responsible for spread of the organism. However, most instances of nasal colonization appear to be associated with infection. This was noted during the studies at Warren Air Force Base [10] and also during the careful epidemiologic observations of Holmes and Williams [11] in the cottage studies. In the latter instance, of 94 individuals who developed illnesses attributed to a specific index case known to harbor hemolytic streptococci, 85% were the result of exposure to nasally colonized index cases and only 15% to those who harbored the organism only in their throats.

Our own studies indicated that it is rare to find nasal colonization in asymptomatic contacts as contrasted to clinically overt individuals, a group much more likely to experience an antibody rise [12]. Positive nose cultures were found more than seven times more frequently in the latter group when compared with the former.

These examples support the contention that carriers do not spread the organism to others nearly as frequently as do individuals who are symptomatic from acute streptococcal pharyngitis.

There is yet another very important consideration when we evaluate the danger of the streptococcal carrier, the risk of development of acute rheumatic fever. In order to reduce the risk of rheumatic fever, the streptococcal infection must be treated to eradicate the organism from the upper respiratory tract. For example, data from Warren Air Force Base indicated that the highest attack rate of acute rheumatic fever (2.8%) occurred with persistence of the homologous strain of group A streptococci after antibiotic therapy, compared to individuals with the appearance of a new strain (an attack rate approximately half as great) or to individuals with negative cultures (only 0.2%) after therapy [13].

However, and this remains a puzzling feature, there are data strongly suggesting that individuals who satisfy our definition of the carrier with persistence of the homologous strain do not often develop rheumatic fever and therefore appear to represent a totally different magnitude of risk. We have indicated that carriers do not experience an antibody response. Data like those of Stetson, for example, tie the magnitude of rise in the antistreptolysin O titer to the attack rate of acute rheumatic fever. Those with ASO titer rises of less than 120 Todd units had an attack rate only one-seventh that of individuals with a rise of 250 or greater Todd units [14]. The less the titer rise, the less the risk of rheumatic fever.

Yet another example is an often-quoted investigation of the attack rate of rheumatic fever in the endemic situation. Evaluation of the data of Siegel, Johnson, and Stollerman from Chicago in the early 1960s is also compatible with the conclusion that the carrier (as defined here) has a lower attack rate of rheumatic fever than the individual with bona fide infection (Table 13–1) [15]. The "normalized" risk of developing rheumatic fever for each of the categories shown in this table has been derived from the original data. Individuals with only sore throat had an attack rate of rheumatic fever of 0.15% in that study. Following normalization of this percentage to a "risk" of 1.0, one can then determine the comparative risk of developing rheumatic fever in those with sore throat plus recovery of group A streptococci as being two and a half times greater. Those with sore throat and a rise in antistreptolysin O titer (bona fide infection) had a six times greater risk. As seen at the bottom of the table, the presence of group A streptococci in the throat, exudative pharyngitis, a rise in ASO titer, and failure to eradicate the organism, surely true infection, resulted in an almost 17 times greater risk of developing rheumatic fever than those with only pharyngitis, or about a six and one-half fold increase in the risk of developing rheumatic fever compared with those who just had group A streptococci present in their throat. These data are also compatible with the concept of a smaller risk for the streptococcal carrier. The authors commented that "acute-phase antibody titers were frequently elevated in this population" [15].

There are a number of other examples that one could cite, but despite the lack of uniform precision and

TABLE 13-1. Relative "Risk Factors" in Patients with Pharyngitis Associated with Development of Rheumatic Fever

| Finding | Number (percentage) | "Normalized" risk of acute rheumatic fever |
|---|---|---|
| Sore throat | 1293 (100) | 1.0 |
| Group A strep recovered | 519 (40) | 2.6X |
| Rise in ASO titer | 228 (18) | 6.0X |
| Exudate pharyngitis | 310 (24) | 4.3X |
| plus positive culture for group A strep | | 6.7X |
| plus rise in ASO titer | | 14.0X |
| plus convalescent "carriage" | | 16.7X |

Source: Modified from Siegel, Johnson, and Stollerman. 1961. NEJM 265:559.

adequately controlled follow-up, it is difficult to ignore the data suggesting that the risk of developing rheumatic fever among carriers is less than among individuals with bona fide streptococcal upper respiratory tract infection. Perhaps we do not need to be so concerned about the carriers.

## WHAT IS APPROPRIATE MANAGEMENT FOR THE CARRIER OR CONTACT?

How can this information influence clinical management of streptococcal carriers and contacts? For the past several years, we have collected data that provide evidence to support ignoring the carrier and that may assist in establishing clinical guidelines.

During an outbreak of group A streptococcal pharyngitis due to an M-58 strain in the semiclosed community of 350 adults and children in St. Paul, we had the opportunity to examine the clinical findings, the epidemiology and the results of antibiotic therapy [16]. Individuals in this study were treated with antibiotics by our study team; compliance was excellent. We found a 25% incidence of antibiotic treatment failures, both following intramuscular benzathine penicillin G and following oral antibiotics (penicillin V or erythromycin). With successive courses of antibiotics given to treatment failures (individuals who continued to harbor the homologous serotype), the rate of failure to eradicate the streptococcus from the throat became even higher, suggesting in retrospect that with each course of therapy we may have selected a higher percentage of carriers.

This unexpectly high treatment failure rate could not be explained by intrafamily spread, by lack of compliance, by antibiotic resistance, or by other factors. Although we did not have complete serologic confirmation, from the available and convalescent sera, it appeared that the treatment failures likely represented a high prevalence of strep-tococcal carriers in this population.

We then undertook a second study to investigate the possibility that carriers were responsible for a high propor-tion of treatment failures. This study was carried out in an endemic situation and included 280 individuals whose mean age was 13 years [17]. Index patients with pharyn-gitis and their asymptomatic family contacts were seen acutely, at three weeks, and eight weeks later; serial bleedings for streptococcal antibody determination were obtained. At the conclusion of the study, we analyzed data from 280 individuals. There were 113 individuals from whom no beta-hemolytic streptococci were isolated on any visit. There were 129 individuals with group A streptococci isolated at their initial visit and 38 with only non-group A streptococci isolated. Treatment success was defined as elimination of the homologous strain without new strains isolated at any of the convalescent visits. Treatment failure was defined as recovery from the upper respiratory tract of group A streptococci of the same serotype at a convalescent visit after completion of antibiotic therapy.

Of the 129 individuals with a positive culture at the first visit, 95 (74%) were bacteriologically cured after their initial visit and 34 were treatment failures. Thirteen of the 34 treatment failures were then successfully retreated, while 21 of 34 required multiple courses of therapy and continued to harbor the homologous strain. Among those treated with intramuscular benzathine penicillin G, we had a 28% failure rate, and we documented a 41% failure rate for those re-ceiving an oral antibiotic that, in almost all instances, was penicillin V.

We evaluated the ASO and anti-DNase B responses of these several groups of individuals. A small percentage (5%) of individuals with no beta-hemolytic streptococci isolated from a throat culture at any visit and those with only non-group A streptococci isolated (5%) showed a sig-nificant rise in antibody titer. Of individuals who were bacteriologic cures at the initial visit or who were one-time treatment failures and then were retreated and cured, 31%

showed a rise in titer. However, of those who were repeated treatment failures, very few (14%) had a rise in
titer. Analysis showed no statistical difference in the
percentage showing a rise among those who were repeated
treatment failures and those who had no streptococci isolated at all. Analysis of the percentage showing a rise in
antibody titer among those who were cured at the initial
visit compared to those who were one-time treatment failures
revealed a significant difference. This strongly suggested
to us that the latter group of individuals was largely composed of carriers.

This could be confirmed by examining the geometric mean
initial antibody titers of these five groups of subjects. The
individuals who were repeated treatment failures had significantly higher initial geometric mean antibody titers than
the other groups. This is compatible with our earlier
studies that indicated that patients who do not show a rise
in antibody titer are likely to have higher initial titers and
are streptococcal upper respiratory tract carriers. This
second way of confirming differences in the immunologic
response to carriers is important because it tends to eliminate or reduce consideration of any suppressive effect of
antibiotics on the immune response.

Since there is always concern about individuals with
asymptomatic streptococcal infection, we examined the
relationship between clinical status and the need for antibiotic retreatment. We divided our patients into three
groups: (1) *clinically overt* patients with complaints of sore
throat plus evidence of either anterior cervical adenitis,
temperature greater than 101° F, pharyngeal or tonsillar
exudate, or pharyngeal injection; (2) *clinically questionable*
patients or family contacts with sore throat or symptoms of
a common cold, but with none of the physical findings
included in the clinically overt category; and (3) *clinically
negative* individuals with no complaints or physical findings
related to infection of the upper respiratory tract. Analysis of the antibody data by clinical status revealed that
individuals with positive cultures for group A streptococci
who were clinically negative rarely (less than 5%) showed a
significant rise in either ASO and/or anti-DNase B titers
and, that their initial geometric mean antibody titers were
much higher than the other two groups. Like patients who
had been treated several times but still harbored the organism, they rarely showed a rise in titer and had high initial
titers.

From these studies we concluded that the incidence of
treatment failure was higher than expected, but that treatment failure patients, especially those who are failures on

more than one occasion, infrequently show a rise in streptococcal antibody titers and have higher geometric mean titers at their initial clinic visit. These immunologic data indicate that this group of patients largely consists of streptococcal carriers.

There are two other studies pertinent to this idea. In the early 1960s Johnson and colleagues carried out a very large study in Denver [18]. Based upon index cases, families were divided into two groups and cultured. All symptomatic patients (index or contact) with positive cultures for group A streptococci were treated. However, in one group (called the prophylaxis group), all asymptomatic individuals with a positive culture were treated while in the "comparison" group no antibiotic treatment was offered to asymptomatic culture-positive individuals. Follow-up took place during the subsequent several months and nonsuppurative sequelae were tabulated. There was no significant difference in nonsuppurative sequelae among those contacts who were treated, when compared with those who were not, suggesting that the risk of nonsuppurative sequelae is not changed by antibiotic treatment of asymptomatic family contacts. In another study, Dunlap and Bergin reported a very low incidence of nonsuppurative sequelae in streptococcal carriers [19]. The figure, incidentally, is quite similar to the figures from the Chicago study by Siegel, Johnson, and Stollerman [15].

Review of the literature, as well as own experience, has led us to believe that the group A streptococcal upper respiratory tract carrier does not usually require repeated courses of antibiotic therapy. In this era of declining rheumatic fever in the United States and most other industrialized countries [20], the obsession with eradicating this organism from the upper respiratory tract of carriers appears to be unnecessary from a practical point of view, even though we do not yet understand the events accompanying the transition from true infection to the carrier state. Why eradication of the organism is necessary in the infected patient and appears not to be necessary in the carrier remains unknown!

While this may be very logical, the clinical problem involved is the accurate prospective identification of the carrier state. We and others have been interested in this for a number of years and while certain clinical findings strongly suggest acute streptococcal infection [21], we still are unable to differentiate consistently and prospectively the symptomatic individual who is a carrier from the symptomatic individual who has bona fide streptococcal infection. Even though it has been reported that approximately one-third of individuals who develop rheumatic fever have experienced asymptomatic infection [22], we believe that it is probably unnecessary to treat asymptomatic contacts even if they have positive cultures. This proposal is supported not only by our data, but also by the studies from Massachusetts [19] and from Denver [18].

From the clinician's standpoint, we might suggest with good reason that individuals who have positive cultures and who are symptomatic be treated with either an appropriate oral antibiotic or intramuscular benzathine penicillin G (Figure 13–3). If asymptomatic after therapy, it seems unnecessary to reculture. If symptomatic following therapy, or if there is an unusual epidemiologic setting, a throat culture can be taken and the patient given an additional course of therapy, for a few of these individuals have *bona fide* infection. We would not, however, continue to reculture and retreat for prolonged periods.

Figure 13–3. Suggestion for antibiotic management of the symptomatic patient with positive culture for group A streptococci in the throat.

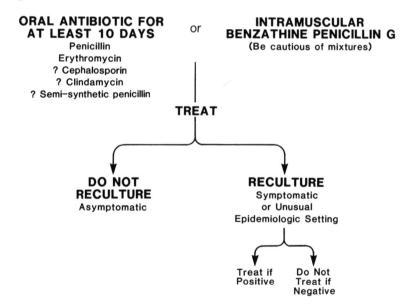

REFERENCES

1. Kaplan, E. L. 1980. The group A streptococcal upper respiratory tract carrier state: An Enigma. *J Pediatr* 97:337.

2. Hamburger, M., Jr., M. J. Green, and V. G. Hamburger. 1945. The problem of the "Dangerous Carrier" of Hemolytic Streptococci. *J Infec Dis* 77:68.

3. Kuttner, A., and E. Krumweide. 1944. Observations on the epidemiology of streptococcal pharyngitis and the relation of streptococcal carriers to the occurrence of outbreaks. *J Clin Invest* 23:139.

4. Kaplan, E. L., F. H. Top, Jr., B. A. Dudding, and L. W. Wannamaker. 1971. Diagnosis of streptococcal pharyngitis: Differentiation of active infection from the carrier state in the symptomatic child. *J Infect Dis* 123:490.

5. Kaplan, E. L., P. Ferrieri, and L. W. Wannamaker. 1974. Comparison of the antibody response to streptococcal cellular and extracellular antigens in acute pharyngitis. *J Pediatr* 84:21.

6. Packer, H., M. B. Arnoult, and D. H. Sprunt. 1956. A study of hemolytic streptococcal infections in relation to antistreptolysin O titer changes in orphanage children. *J Pediatr* 48:545.

7. Mozziconacci, P., C. L. Gerbeaux, R. Caravano, S. Gerbeaux, J. Labonde, S. Rahman, F. Rabcynska, E. Orssaud, and P. Virolleau. 1961. A study of group A hemolytic streptococcus Carriers Among School Children. II. Significance of the findings. *Acta Paediatr Scand* 50:33.

8. Krause, R. M., and C. H. Rammelkamp, Jr. 1962. Studies of the carrier state following infection with group A streptococci. II. Infectivity of streptococci isolated during acute pharyngitis and during the carrier state. *J Clin Invest* 41:575.

9. Coburn, A. F., and R. H. Pauli. 1941. The interaction of host and bacterium in the development of communicability by *Streptococcus haemolyticus*. *J Exp Med* 73:551.

10. Wannamaker, L. W. 1954. The Epidemiology of Streptococcal Infections. In *Streptococcal Infections,* 157. M. McCarty, ed. New York: Columbia University Press.

11. Holmes, M. C., and R. E. O. Williams. 1958. Streptococcal infections among children in a residential home. II. Potential sources of infection for individuals. *J Hyg* 56:62.

12. Kaplan, E. L., R. Couser, A. S. Gastanaduy, and

B. B. Huwe. N.d. Unpublished observations.

13. Catanzaro, F. J., C. H. Rammelkamp, and R. Chamovitz. 1958. Prevention of rheumatic fever by treatment of streptococcal infection. II. Factors responsible for failures. *New Engl J Med* 259:51.

14. Stetson, C. A., Jr. 1954. The Relation of Antibody Response to Rheumatic Fever. In *Streptococcal Infections*, 208. M. McCarty, ed. New York: Columbia University Press.

15. Siegel, A. C., E. E. Johnson, and G. H. Stollerman. 1961. Controlled studies of streptococcal pharyngitis in a pediatric population. I. Factors related to the attack rate of rheumatic fever. *New Engl J Med* 265:559.

16. Gastanaduy, A. S., E. L. Kaplan, B. B. Huwe, C. McKay, and L. W. Wannamaker. 1980. Failure of penicillin to eradicate group A streptococci during an outbreak of pharyngitis. *Lancet* 2:498.

17. Kaplan, E. L., A. S. Gastanaduy, and B. B. Huwe. 1981. The role of the carrier in treatment failures after antibiotic therapy for group A streptococci in the upper respiratory tract. *J Lab Clin Med* 98:326.

18. Johnson, S., C. W. Streamer, and P. W. Williams. 1964. An evaluation of a streptococcal control program. *Am J Public Health* 54:487.

19. Dunlap, M. B., and J. W. Bergin. 1973. Subsequent health of former carriers of hemolytic streptococci. *NY State J Med* 73:1875.

20. Strasser, T. 1978. Rheumatic fever and rheumatic heart disease in the 1970's. *WHO Chron* 32:18.

21. Wannamaker, L. W. Chapter 4.

22. Gordis, L., A. Lilienfeld, and R. Rodriguez. 1964. Studies in the epidemiology and preventability of rheumatic fever. I. Demographic factors and the incidence of acute attacks. *J Chronic Dis* 21:645.

# 14

# The Role of Models for Medical Decisions: Algorithms and Decision Analysis

## *Alvan R. Feinstein, M.D.*

I would have hoped to have been invited here as a loyal alumnus of the University of Rheumatic Fever, who spent happy years studying and working there, and who could reminisce about undergraduate capers, while joining in the discussion of problems created by a declining enrollment of patients at my alma mater. We are not sure how much of the reduced incidence of rheumatic fever today is due to better diagnosis of other diseases that formerly masqueraded under the rheumatic-fever label, and how much is due to the role of antibiotics in preventing or eradicating streptococcal infections. We do know, however, that rheumatic fever now occurs infrequently enough (in technologically well-developed countries) to warrant the current reappraisal of our approaches to the etiologic streptococcal culprit.

My assignment in this conference, however, is to focus on work I have done in my postgraduate career. As an excellent university, Rheumatic Fever prepared me for many challenges that waited in the world beyond. The ones I have been asked to discuss today are the models used for making medical decisions. I shall try to be clear and dispassionate in describing the models, but my lack of enthusiasm for some of them may sometimes escape during editorial comments.

In contemplating models for decision making, clinicians may focus their thoughts on the models, rather than on the decisions to which the models are applied. I shall organize my remarks according to the fundamental issues, which are the decisions. There are two main types of decisions in clinical practice: intellectual decisions and action decisions.

Intellectual decisions are what we do when we arrive at a conclusion about a diagnostic title for a patient's ailment, a belief about etiology or pathogenesis of the ailment, or a prognostic estimate about what is going to happen. These are intellectual decisions, because they involve reasoning alone, and they occur after all the evidence has been assembled. The decision itself produces a name, an idea, or a prediction, but not something that can directly happen to a patient and that can produce benefit or harm.

Action decisions are what we do in choosing and performing the technologic tests that provide evidence for the intellectual decisions, and in recommending and giving therapy that may be used remedially to change something that has already happened or prophylactically to prevent something that has not yet occurred. The action decisions are the ones that produce interventions, directly imposed on the patient, that can sometimes be beneficial and sometimes not. The technologic tests yield valuable information, but may create hazardous complications; and the therapeutic activities can sometimes kill or maim rather than prevent, cure, or relieve.

To understand the models that have been proposed for these decisions, we need first to separate the two main types.

INTELLECTUAL DECISIONS

Etiology

For intellectual decisions about etiology, such as the conclusion that the Group A streptococcus causes rheumatic fever or the recent proposal that coffee drinking may cause pancreatic cancer, the models depend on an intricate array of experimental and observational evidence, often interpreted with complex statistical strategies. To stay within my alloted time, I shall not discuss these complexities.

Prognosis

I shall also give relatively short shrift to models used for decisions about prognosis. The models here are mainly mathematical, with multivariate statistical analyses producing numerical scores, such as the Apgar Score, or clustered categories, such as the Stages I, II, and III of a TNM staging system for cancer. The Apgar Score and TNM staging system were actually formed in an old "cottage industry" called *clinical judgment*, but the new mathematical models of prognosis are produced in a modern, automated, computerized "factories." An example of one of these models is called multiple linear regression. It takes the data expressed in values of variables such as $x_1$, for age, $x_2$ for *severity of symptoms*, and so on. As the computer crunches the numbers, the model assigns the weighting coefficients $b_1, b_2$, and so on, for each variable. What emerges is an expression such as $y = b_0 + b_1x_1 + b_2x_2 + b_3x_3 +, \ldots$ where y is the prognostic prediction. Thus, when a new patient comes along, we can predict prognosis by entering his values of the appropriate variables into an equation that may look like: Expected survival time = 6.1 - 0.07 (age) - 0.32 (severity of symptoms) + .48 (gender) + 0.02 (hematocrit) +. . . . It may not resemble prognostic reasoning, but it is a lovely model.

Diagnosis

I shall spend a good bit of time on diagnostic decisions, because one of the models (called *Bayes Theorem*) has become quite fashionable, and often appears in medical literature. For diagnostic decisions, iatromathematicians have developed models that offer formulas for interpreting and using the data of diagnostic tests, but the model builders seldom indicate that there are three different types of diagnostic tests: definitive, contributory, and surrogate.

A *definitive test*, such as a liver biopsy or glucose tolerance test, requires no special formulas or interpretations. It provides the "gold standard" evidence of diagnosis. The test itself shows that the patient either does or does not have hepatitis or diabetes mellitus. A *contributory test*, such as evidence of antecedent streptococcal infection in the diagnosis of rheumatic fever, is joined with other evidence in decisions about whether the patient fulfills the demands contained in such stipulations as the Jones Diagnostic Criteria. The contributory test, however, is not used alone to make a diagnosis or to substitute for the definitive evidence.

A *surrogate test*, such as carcinoembryonic antigen (CEA) in the diagnosis of colon cancer or VDRL for syphilis, is used as a substitute for the definitive evidence. This surrogate role is what has inspired the artistry of the mathematical models. The models are used to help decide how accurately the surrogate test does its job. The job assignment can give a surrogate test one of three different roles. In *screening*, a surrogate test is usually given during a campaign or mass populational survey, and is received by people in whom there is no suspicion of disease. A surrogate test is also used for a type of screening that is more appropriately called *case finding*. A case-finding test is ordered, again without suspicion of the associated disease, in a medical setting as part of the routine "workup" for patients who have sought care for other reasons. The surrogate test may also be used for *differential diagnosis* in patients whose manifestations evoke suspicion of the target disease, but in these circumstances, an efficient clinician will usually rely on a more powerful contributory or definitive test. Thus, to diagnose a patient who has had rectal bleeding or a change in stool diameter, the doctor will usually order sigmoidoscopy and/or a barium enema, and not just a CEA test.

The basic intellectual flaw in our use of surrogate tests is that they are almost always first developed and tested for accuracy in patients hospitalized with overt manifestations that suggest the disease, and the "test group" contains roughly equal proportions of diseased and non-diseased patients. The tests are then applied, however, for screening and case-finding in the community, to people who do not have such manifestations, and to a population whose prevalence of disease is much lower than in the contrived "test group."

This shift has two major consequences. Scientifically, we do not know whether the test responds the same way to give the same results in people with overt manifestations as it does in those who are symptomless. Statistically, the diagnostic accuracy of the test will be dramatically altered when it is transferred from its hospital origin to the community. The mathematical models for diagnosis are aimed exclusively at the statistical problem; and the scientific problem—although quite important—has been generally ignored. I shall maintain that tradition.

To demonstrate the statistical problem, we can use the data in Table 14–1, which gives a set of hypothetical results for the hospital groups receiving Alvanol, a surrogate test for a particular disease. When used in 100 diseased patients, the test had a sensitivity of 95%; and its specificity was 97% in the 100 nondiseased controls. When this table is viewed not vertically, but horizontally (the way a clinician would interpret the results), the data translate into an accuracy of 97% when the test result is

TABLE 14-1.  Hypothetical Results of Alvanol Test: Hospital Groups

| Test result | Diseased patients | Nondiseased controls | Total |
|---|---|---|---|
| Positive | 95 | 3 | 98 |
| Negative | 5 | 97 | 102 |
| Total | 100 | 100 | 200 |

Sensitivity = 95/100 = 95%
Specificity = 97/100 = 97%
Accuracy for positive result = 95/98 = 97%
Accuracy for negative result = 97/102 = 95%

positive and 95% when it is negative.  It thus seems like an excellent test.

Table 14–2, however, shows what happens when Alvanol is applied outside of the hospital in a community screening population where the disease occurs at a rate of 1 per 100. Thus, of 10,000 people in the community, 100 have the disease and 9900 do not.  The test will still have its sensitivity of 95% and specificity of 97%.  Its accuracy for a negative result will be improved—up to almost 100%.  The accuracy for a positive result, however, has been dramatically lowered to 24%.  The test will therefore yield a false-positive conclusion, which, if heeded, will evoke an unnecessary workup in about three-fourths of all people with positive results.  Because of the high accuracy when negative, the test might be splendid for ruling out the disease, but the price we pay in using this test to find disease in the community is a large number of false-positive signals.

A thoughtful clinician would promptly understand this distinction about use of the test and could readily see the difference from an inspection of these two tables; but just in case he has missed the point, a mathematical model has been developed to use sensitivity, specificity, and (especially) prevalence of the disease for calculating the accuracy of a positive or negative result.  To guard against the threat of clarity if the formula were presented in simple algebra, the ideas are converted, as shown in Table 14–3, into symbols of conditional probability, organized in an

TABLE 14-2.  Hypothetical Results of Alvanol Test: Screening Population

| Test result | Diseased patients | Nondiseased controls | Total |
|---|---|---|---|
| Positive | 95 | 297 | 392 |
| Negative | 5 | 9603 | 9608 |
| Total | 100 | 9900 | 10,000 |

Sensitivity = 95/100 = 95%
Specificity = 9603/9900 = 97%
Accuracy for positive result = 95/392 = 24%
Accuracy for negative result = 9603/9608 $\cong$ 100%

TABLE 14-3.  Formulations for Diagnostic Accuracy of Positive Result

| | Symbols | Formula |
|---|---|---|
| Simple Algebra | $v$ = Sensitivity<br>$f$ = Specificity<br>$d$ = Prevalence of Disease | $\dfrac{vd}{vd + [(1 - f)(1 - d)]}$ |
| Conditional probability; Bayes Theorem | $P(S\|D)$ = Sensitivity<br>$P(\overline{S}\|\overline{D})$ = Specificity<br>$P(D)$ = Prevalence<br>$P(\overline{D})$ = 1-Prevalence | $\dfrac{P(S\|D)\,P(D)}{P(S\|D)\,P(D) + P(S\|D)\,P(D)}$ |

appropriately inscrutable conglomeration, and labelled with the majestic eponym of *Bayes Theorem.*

Since the conveners of the conference have wisely limited my time, you will be spared many other details and delicacies that might be added to the mathematical excitement. I shall summarize the Bayesian decision-making model by stating that the fundamental scientific fallacy of assuming that sensitivity and specificity are constant in all parts of the clinical spectrum, and the absence of a resemblance to the way clinicians really reason diagnostically have kept this model from achieving a pragmatic clinical acceptance comparable to the enormous attraction the model has held for investigators and editors of medical journals.

## ACTION DECISIONS

With these preliminaries completed, we can now turn to my main event: the two principal models used for action decisions. Since most of the existing models are aimed at therapy rather than diagnostic workups, I shall confine my discussion to therapeutic decisions. The decision-making principles remain the same if the models are applied to the ordering of diagnostic tests.

### Algorithms

The first type of model for action decisions provides a set of instructions or guidelines that stipulate someone's clinical judgment, but there is no demonstration of the actual reasoning or justification. The model simply tells a person what to do. Models of this type have often been called protocols, and used to give paramedical personnel instructions about how to manage patients with urinary symptoms, sore throats, low back pain, and other common medical complaints. The instructions can be expressed in a verbal sequence, somewhat like a cookbook recipe; but since many different contingencies may be encountered, the instructions require many different branchings to deal with each contingency. Because a computer program also contains a series of sequential decisions that are made for each encountered contingency, the nomenclature and symbols of computer programming have been used effectively for this purpose.

Thus, the instructions are sometimes given in the form of *decision tables*, which resemble the format of a crossword puzzle, or as *decision trees*, which are also called *algorithms* and which are visually displayed as *flow charts*. Figure 14–1 shows an elementary algorithm or flow chart, indicating the customary instructions to be given to a driver approaching a traffic light. If the light is green, the driver is told to go. If the light is not green, the next decision is whether the light is yellow. If the answer to this question is yes, the driver is told to slow down and make a new decision later. If the light is not yellow, it can be presumed to be red and the driver is told to stop.

Figure 14–1.  Traffic light algorithm

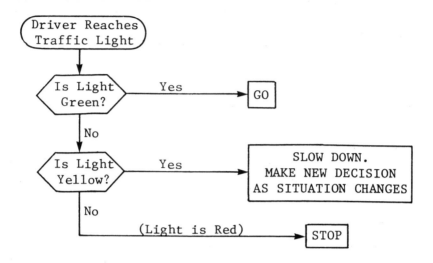

Decision Analysis

Although algorithms show the conclusions of the reasoning, they do not indicate the rational process itself. The attempt to demonstrate a rational process, weighing the different risks and benefits of therapy, is provided by a model called *decision analysis*, which is the subject of the rest of my discussion.

The basic strategy of decision analysis in choosing therapy for a particular clinical situation is as follows:

1. Prepare a flow chart or other diagram that shows the complete sequential pattern of all possible decisions and all possible outcomes for each decision.
2. Establish a utility value for each possible outcome.
3. Assign probabilities for the likelihood of occurrence of each possible outcome.
4. Calculate scores for the products of the values for probabilities and utilities. Add the scores appropriately.
5. Choose the decision that has the best score.

Since clinical examples always become quite complicated, the simplest way I know to illustrate this process is by showing an act of culinary judgment, called the "rotten egg" decision.

Let us assume that five good eggs have been broken into a bowl for making an omelet. A sixth egg, which may be rotten, is unbroken and available. We must decide what to do with this unbroken egg. We can take three possible actions: (A) Break the egg directly into the bowl containing the other five eggs; (B) break it into a saucer and inspect it; or (C) throw the egg away without inspecting its contents.

Table 14–4 shows a tabular version of the algorithm containing each possible action and outcome. Let us first consider Action A—breaking the egg directly into the bowl containing the other five eggs. If the new egg is good, we have a six-egg omelet. If the new egg is rotten, everything is ruined and we have no omelet. Next, consider the tactic of breaking the egg into a saucer and checking it. Regardless of the result, we will have an extra saucer to wash. If the egg is good, we add it to the omelet; if bad, we throw it away. Finally, we can throw the egg away, without inspection. We would then be left with a five-egg omelet, but with the chance of having wasted a potentially good egg.

Now that we have contemplated each possible decision and outcome, our next step is to establish "utility values" for the outcomes. To do so, let us assume that eggs cost 10 cents apiece and that the cost of washing a saucer is 1 cent. With outcome I, there is no loss. With outcome II, we lose the entire investment of $0.60 in the six eggs. With outcome III, we lose $0.01 (to wash the saucer). With outcome IV, we lose $0.11 (an egg and a saucer-wash). For either outcome V and VI, we lose $0.10.

We next need to know the probability or likelihood for the occurrence of each outcome. In this example, everything depends on whether the egg is good or rotten. Let us assume there is one chance in ten that the egg is rotten. Thus, the probability of a good egg is 0.9 and the probability of a rotten egg is 0.1.

Our next step is to multiply the probabilities and utilities to get a potential score for each possible action. For Action A, the score for outcome 1 is $0.9 \times 0$ (since there is no loss); and the score for outcome II is $0.1 \times (-0.60) = -0.06$. The net score for Action A is thus $0 - 0.06 = -0.06$. For Action B, the net score is $(0.9)(-0.01) + (0.1)(-0.11) = -0.02$. For Action C, the net score is $(0.9)(-0.10) + (0.1)(-0.10) = -0.10$.

The result indicates that Action B is the best thing to do. It has the least net loss associated with it. The analysis also suggests that the worst thing to do is to throw the egg away unexamined.

TABLE 14-4. Actions and Outcomes for Rotten-Egg Dilemma

| Identity of action | Action | State of egg | Outcome | Identity of outcome |
|---|---|---|---|---|
| A | Break into bowl | Good | Six-egg omelet; no loss | I |
| | | Rotten | Five good eggs ruined; no omelet | II |
| B | Break into saucer | Good | Six-egg omelet; saucer to wash | III |
| | | Rotten | Five-egg omelet; saucer to wash | IV |
| C | Discard egg | Good | Five-egg omelet; good egg wasted | V |
| | | Rotten | Five-egg omelet | VI |

If we now stop to evaluate the principles that produced the score for this "worst" decision, we can begin to see the real problems of using decision analysis. Is throwing away the egg really the worst thing to do? You might want to argue that it is not, and that the worst thing to do is to break the egg directly into the bowl. Throwing the egg away leaves us assured of having at least a five-egg omelet; whereas breaking the egg directly into the bowl makes us take the chance of ruining everything and having no omelet at all.

The difficulties here are that the original model we established was incomplete. The general plan of sequential strategy did not include provision for several other contingencies and for other issues and values that were not examined. Are more eggs available? If so, are there enough to make another six-egg omelet? Is there some method to determine whether an egg is rotten without breaking and inspecting it? If so, how accurate is the method and is it readily available? Will a five-egg omelet be satisfactory, although smaller, or must the omelet contain at least six eggs? After all, if we can readily get as many other eggs as we need, we might be willing to risk the loss of the entire omelet; but if no other eggs are available, the total waste of the available eggs might be a catastrophe whose painful consequences have a loss value of much more than $0.60. If we can easily and confidently determine whether the egg is rotten before it is broken, the rest of our plans would be substantially altered. As a different possibility, suppose the omelet must contain at least six eggs, because anything smaller would be unacceptable. In this circumstance, if no other eggs are available, we would have to break the potentially rotten egg directly into the bowl because this action is the only possible way to get a six-egg omelet. Even if the egg is rotten, the risk of no omelet would be equal to that of having only an unacceptable five-egg omelet.

### Designing a complete algorithm

The examples just noted help illustrate the problems of creating an algorithm, estimating the probabilities, and establishing the utilities that will constitute a complete, accurate model of the decision under analysis. The first main problem is the necessity for specifying the total algorithmic plan, containing provision for every contingency that is pertinent.

If making an omelet requires an algorithm as complicated as the one just discussed, what must be the complexity of the plan that includes all possible conditions, actions, and outcomes for a decision about a patient's care? For example, suppose we need to decide whether to administer an antibiotic to a patient with a sore throat. We might easily be able to establish a simple algorithm in which the decision depends only on certain clinical characteristics of the history and physical examination. Such an algorithm, however, would be crude and incomplete. It would contain no provision for such contingencies as: the possibility of withholding treatment until we learn the results of throat culture; the patient's ability to return for another visit after the throat culture results became known; the likelihood that the patient would actually return for such a visit; the patient's ability to purchase a prescribed oral antibiotic; the likelihood that the patient would actually buy it; and the likelihood that the patient, having bought it, would actually take it as prescribed. These are but a few of the many contingencies that a thoughtful clinician thinks about when engaged in decision making for the sore-throat situation—and the citation of all possible contingencies would lead to an algorithm of enormous complexity.

### Establishing probabilities

Assuming that a truly complete plan could be developed to list all possible contingencies, we would next be confronted with specifying the probability values for the contingencies. To calculate the scores required for an analytic decision, a precise quantitative value must be stipulated for each of the possibilities. For the omelet decision, the only probability we needed to list was the likelihood that the egg was rotten. Had the planning algorithm been more complete, however, we might have had to determine probabilities for such events as the chances that other eggs would be available or that the quality of the egg could be determined before it is broken.

When we try to list all of the probabilities that require specification for a clinical rather than a culinary decision, the task quickly leaves the realm of quantitative science because there is no way to get reliable data for most of the necessary probability values. Some of the probabilities require purely clinical information, but the data exist only in crude forms. For example, we might be able to scan the medical literature and find an exact value for the probability that a child with a sore throat has a beta-hemolytic streptococcal infection. The information in the literature would not be detailed enough, however, to indicate the exact probability of such an infection in the sore throat of a 9-year-old girl with 2+ enlarged tonsils, exudate, cervical adenopathy, cough, no fever, and a history of frequent previous sore throats that were negative on culture for streptococcus. Yet the latter probability is the one we would need to know for the formal process of decision analysis to receive an appropriate quantitative structure.

Another set of probabilities depends on nonclinical information that seldom has a precise quantitative basis. What is the likelihood that the 9-year-old girl will faithfully take a ten-day course of penicillin? Suppose we guess it to be *highly likely*. Is *highly likely* to be represented by a probability value of 0.9, 0.95, 0.85, or even 0.75?

Assuming that the probability values can somehow be successfully established, however, a third set of problems still remains. These problems, which arise from the selection of utility values, are the ultimate, insurmountable obstacle to the realistic application of quantitatively measured decision analysis.

### Choice of utility values

For the omelet decision, we used only two "utility values": the cost of the eggs and the cost of washing an extra saucer. If the original algorithm were more complex, however, we would have had to consider many other aspects of "utility." These further considerations would produce a series of formidable or insurmountable problems.

The first kind of problem arises from the difficulty of determining the relative magnitude of complicated utility values. In Action B, for example, we could readily learn the cost of an egg, but how did we decide that the cost of washing an extra saucer was 1 cent? To make this decision by quantitative calculation, we would have to determine the cost of soap, water, human labor, and perhaps some additional potential losses, such as the risk of breaking the saucer during its usage. Although the information and calculations might eventually produce the utility value of 1 cent, the prerequisite efforts would be extremely cumbersome. If many such calculations were needed, the advantages of a decision-analysis procedure might be negated by the amount of work needed to get the utility values.

The second kind of problem in utility values is much more serious than the difficulty of cumbersome calculations. The problem arises in the many circumstances in which a utility value cannot be calculated. For example, consider the possible adverse consequences of Action A. If the entire omelet were ruined and if no other eggs were available, the total loss would be more than the 60 cents paid for the six eggs. The total concept of "utility" would have to include not only the cook's despair, frustration, or sheer hunger in not having an anticipated omelet, but also the possible rage or anger of the cook's spouse. Similarly, if we followed plan C and emerged with a five-egg omelet, the total loss would be more than the 10 cents paid for the discarded egg. There would also be the disappointment or deprivation of having to eat an undersized omelet.

For a total utility score to be calculated, these despairs or disappointments would need to be expressed and incorporated into the individual utility values. These expressions can be attained only after performance of two separate judgments: first, the magnitude of the despair or disappointment must be graded or ranked; and second, the graded rating must be converted into the type of unit used for the dimension of the other utility values. Thus, to complete the array of utilities for Action A, we would have to determine the degree of frustration (or hunger) incurred by the deprivation of an expected omelet. Next, after this degree is determined, we must convert it into monetary units so that it will be cited in terms commensurate with those of the other utility values. Proceeding along these lines, we might arrive at the value of $2.00 as the utility debit for the loss of the omelet.

When utility values must be assigned in clinical situations, this type of problem is insurmountable. What is the numerically measurable "utility" to a family of a peaceful, nonprotracted death for a relative? What is the utility of avoiding an unwanted pregnancy? What is the utility of avoiding a severe penicillin reaction? None of these questions can be answered in any standard manner and none of the answers can readily be cited in monetary (or other dimensional) units.

We thus come to the final obstacle that militates against the hope that utility values can ever be set or used in a realistic manner. Who chooses the utility values? Are they to be established by doctors, patients, or "society"? Different decision makers may set dramatically different values for the same outcome. For example, a newly married, childless 40-year-old woman may place an extremely high value on whatever efforts are needed to help her become pregnant and carry to term. A doctor, as a different decision maker, may feel the risks are not worth the benefits, but might be willing to accede to her request. A third choice might come from a panel of economists, who allegedly represent "society" in setting policy for a national health program. The economists, evaluating the potentially high costs of care, may establish so negative a value for the utility that the pregnancy is strongly discouraged.

Because dimensional units, often monetary, ultimately become the common numerical expression for the kind of cost/benefit appraisals that create quantitative utility measurements, we would need to set a numerical value on all of the diverse joys and sorrows, gratifications and frustrations that can occur in human life. The difficulties both of establishing such numbers and (in a free society) of choosing the number-fixers become insurmountable obstacles for anyone who seriously wants to make routine use of quantitative decision analysis in the clinical practice of medicine.

### The role of sensitivity analysis

The many bright people, like Drs. Tompkins and Pantell, who have been working in this field are well aware of these problems and complaints; and so they have created an apparent escape hatch called *sensitivity analysis*. It works as follows: If you are uncertain about a particular probability, choose a range of possibilities. If uncertain about a particular utility value, choose a range of reasonable extremes. After establishing these ranges for each uncertain value, recalculate all the scores, using all combinations of extremes in these new ranges. If necessary, use a computer to check all the possible vicissitudes of scores for all the possible ranges.

When these calculations are finished, if the decision chosen previously still emerges with the best final score, stick to it. If not, make suitable appraisals and adaptations.

This strategy certainly provides a flexible approach. The main problem is that we may still wind up using old-fashioned clinical judgment to evaluate the disagreements in scores and to reach a decision.

## PERSONAL CONCLUSIONS

Although a formal, quantitatively measured decision analysis becomes destroyed by the insuperable obstacles of having to guess probabilities and conjure utilities, I believe the first part of the process—preparing algorithms or sequential outlines of possible actions and outcomes—makes a valuable contribution to clinical reasoning. When forced to contemplate this pathway, physicians and patients will fully outline what must be contemplated for each decision. The outcomes can usually be narrowed to the few that are most important, and they can then be approached with reasoning that is sometimes called "risk aversion." I use the name "chagrin factor" for the way this principle is employed.

According to this principle, we want to avoid those things that will make us feel particularly chagrined if they occur. We therefore tend to avoid any pathway in the flow chart that might let these events occur in a way that imposes chagrin. Thus, a patient with a group A streptococcal infection might still get rheumatic fever even if treated, but we would feel chagrin if we left him untreated and he developed it. We therefore decide to treat. (This is somewhat like establishing a utility value of minus infinity for that outcome.)

We would also feel chagrin if the patient developed an adverse reaction to the treatment, but did not have a strep infection. We therefore get a throat culture, using it somewhat like the saucer for checking the possibly rotten egg. In an era of effective oral therapy, if the patient is reliable, we can start oral treatment promptly, taking a reduced chance of adverse reaction because the treatment is oral. If the culture comes back negative, we can stop the treatment. If the culture is positive, treatment is continued.

The chagrin factor is an important determinant of clinical decisions, and it is often evoked by risks as low as one in

100. Thus, the risk of rheumatic fever after a strep infection is roughly about 0.01. The risk of poliomyelitis in the days before the vaccine was probably about 0.01 or less. Nevertheless, to avoid chagrin, we vaccinate everyone against polio and most clinicians would want to treat strep infections when they are detected. Since women were having babies quite successfully long before God created obstetricians, we know that most babies will emerge successfully if someone merely hangs around to catch them. Nevertheless, there is a risk of about 0.01 that a major problem may occur at the time of delivery. To manage that problem on that one occasion in a hundred, most people prefer to have a competent obstetrician available at all deliveries.

Although I can sometimes admire and applaud the majestic models of the iatromathematicians, I strongly suspect that none of the probabilities, utilities, sensitivity analyses, and other quantitative calculations will ever replace the important judgmental process that produces decisions by answering the question: What will give me chagrin—and how can I best avoid it?

# 15

# Developing, Testing, and Evaluating Algorithms for Managing Pharyngitis

*Richard K. Tompkins, M.D.*

During the past decade there has been a serious attempt to analyze medical decisions in a systematic, rigorous, and objective manner. The goals of the clinicians involved in this endeavor have been to establish a quantitative basis for diagnostic and therapeutic decisions; to define what is effective in patient care; and to identify important areas of ignorance, so that new knowledge can be sought that will have direct impact on the care patients receive. More recently, because of the explosion in medical care costs, cost-effectiveness analysis and the study of medical decisions have been integrated.

Some of the original work that preceded the expansion of interest in decision theory among clinicians was directed at elucidating formal decision rules (algorithms or protocols) that could be used to teach nonphysicians to manage common illnesses and to monitor the effectiveness of these providers in this role. Because sore throat is such a common symptom, it was an inevitable choice for early attempts to define explicit rules for its diagnosis and management. Since this symposium is concerned with pharyngitis and its sequelae, I want to use the development of algorithms for this disease as a case study in medical decision making. Additionally, I hope to convince you that algorithms are a practical method to standardize treatment, in a manner that emphasizes cost-effective, up-to-date practices.

Algorithms, or protocols, are explicit descriptions of steps to be taken in managing a patient with a particular problem. The algorithm specifies the history, physical examination, and laboratory data that should be collected; and it uses those data to prescribe therapy, further diagnostic tests, or referrals. The rules that the algorithm uses—usually branching logic or discriminant scores—allow management to be individualized for each patient but still constrain the universe of management options. In practice, the provider using an algorithm employs it as a "guidance system" to help improve efficiency and effectiveness, but he still maintains the option to deviate from the algorithm instructions, if appropriate for an individual patient.

The algorithm "system" that my colleagues and I have experimented with during the past 12 years consists of the algorithm logic itself, a checklist form that serves as a data-recording device, and a group of computer programs that store, manipulate, and retrieve the data from the checklists. The development of a clinical algorithm has generally been carried out in five sequential stages:

1. A clinical problem is chosen that is common enough to warrant the effort (for example, sore throat).
2. A list of the diseases that cause the problem is prepared and categorized by their seriousness and incidence and by the effectiveness of medical intervention upon their prevention or prognosis. Rare problems or those that are unaffected by medical care usually are omitted.
3. The clinical data needed to diagnose or treat these diseases are defined and their sensitivity and specificity determined, if possible. Then a decision tree is constructed that defines how these data are to be used.
4. The algorithm and its logic are evaluated in controlled clinical trials, gathering data that permit refinement of the logic and testing many of the data elements for reproducibility, sensitivity, specificity, and predictive value.
5. The evaluation data are used to redefine the algorithm and improve its effectiveness, efficiency, and ease of use. Then the new algorithm is retested in a more limited clinical trial.

ALGORITHM DEVELOPMENT

Several sore throat management algorithms were developed to be part of a more general algorithm for acute upper respiratory illness (URI). Originally, three respiratory illness algorithms (URI, ear problems, and cough) were developed empirically—based on clinical judgment and literature review—to mimic "good medical practice" and to be used specifically by physician's assistants [1]. As a result of compiling data on the medical care resulting from using these algorithms in many different practices and in thousands of patient encounters, it became clear that the algorithms relied excessively on diagnostic tests, required too much physician involvement, and were not efficient enough. We recognized that a new, simpler algorithm could be written that would be more cost-effective and would not sacrifice safety, quality, or patient satisfaction.

To define which data would be useful for the new algorithm, 5,000 adult patients were studied in a controlled clinical setting where an extensive, standardized data base could be collected [2]. Multiple statistical analyses were performed to identify unproductive logic, high-cost or low-yield diagnostic tests, and causes for unnecessary physician involvement. All history and physical examination data were tested for inter-observer reproducibility.

Because sore throat was the most prevalent URI symptom in the patient populations we studied, we also performed a formal cost-benefit analysis of pharyngitis management and acute rheumatic fever prevention [3]. This study suggested that patients with at least a 20% risk of a positive throat culture for group A streptococci should be treated with penicillin immediately. Conversely, those patients with a 5% or less risk did not require either a throat culture for diagnosis or treatment with penicillin. Based on this analysis, the goal of the new sore throat algorithm was to assign patients to one of three categories:

- High risk (risk 20% or greater): These patients received penicillin treatment without a diagnosis being confirmed by a throat culture.
- Medium risk (risk 5%–20%): These patients received penicillin only if the throat culture was positive.
- Low risk (risk 5% or less): These patients were neither cultured nor treated.

Prior to writing the new sore throat algorithm, we analyzed the reproducibility, sensitivity, and specificity of all the history and physical examination data useful in evaluating patients for possible streptococcal pharyngitis [4]. We found that no single clinical finding can distinguish between streptococcal and nonstreptococcal disease (Table 15–1) and that some findings are not very reproducible. We have defined several algorithms for adults and

TABLE 15-1. Clinical Predictors of Streptococcal—Positive Patients

| Finding | Inter-MD kappa value in populations of: | | Sensitivity* | Specificity* | Predictive Value* |
| --- | --- | --- | --- | --- | --- |
| | Adults | Children | | | |
| Random choice | 0.00 | 0.00 | 0.50 | 0.50 | 0.10 |
| Sore throat | 0.74 | 0.55 | 1.00 | 0.00 | 0.00 |
| Strep exposure | 0.12 | 0.64 | 0.25 | 0.88 | 0.27 |
| Absence of cough | 0.87 | 0.81 | 0.83 | 0.48 | 0.22 |
| Absence of rhinorrhea | 0.75 | 0.60 | 0.73 | 0.48 | 0.20 |
| Fever $\geq$ 38.3° C | 0.94 | -- | 0.17 | 0.94 | 0.33 |
| Pharyngeal erythema | 0.36 | 0.11 | 0.98 | 0.16 | 0.17 |
| Pharyngeal exudate | 0.36 | 0.59 | 0.47 | 0.79 | 0.29 |
| Enlarged cervical nodes | 0.02 | 0.12 | 0.94 | 0.27 | 0.19 |

*In adult patients with sore throat as a presenting symptom.

196

children with sore throats, each of which has some differences in the medical logic, reflecting differences in patient population characteristics and different clinical priorities [2,5,6]. For example, the algorithm in Figure 15-1 was designed for use in a large, acute minor illness clinic in an Army medical center where reduction in cost was an important priority [2]. The algorithm in Figure 15-2 was for a medium-sized HMO that wanted to handle as many patients as possible by telephone [5]. Each of these algorithms was developed using Bayesian analysis of data from each clinic's patients, collected by their own providers. Thus the algorithms are "tailor made" to a specific patient population, group of providers, and set of operational priorities.

## CLINICAL EVALUATION OF THE ALGORITHM

To show that the algorithm in Figure 15-1 was as safe and effective as traditional care, we compared the results when physician's assistants managed patients using the algorithm with management by internists who did not use the algorithm [2]. The patient populations were statistically similar and thus comparable. The internists' care became the "gold standard"; prior to the study, these physicians had agreed among themselves that their goal was to treat with penicillin all patients whose throat cultures were positive. Therefore, during the algorithm validation we obtained throat culture from most patients, even though the physician's assistants used them to make treatment decisions only when specified by the algorithm. The results of the comparative study are shown in Table 15-2 and can be summarized as follows:

- Internists treated fewer patients with streptococcal pharyngitis with penicillin than did the physician's assistants who used the algorithm (85% versus 91%). This difference is not statistically significant.
- The algorithm led to prescribing antibiotic treatment significantly ($p < 0.05$) more often for patients with negative throat cultures than did the physicians (31% vs 26%).

The data collected during this study also confirmed that the sore throat algorithm selected patients with a predictable risk of having streptococcal pharyngitis. Of the 94 patients in the high-risk group, 21% had positive cultures; of the 188 patients in the moderate risk group, 9% had positive cultures; and in the low risk group, comprising 263

Figure 15–1.  Sore Throat Strategy

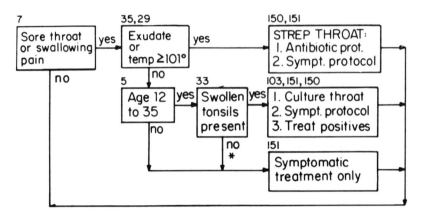

Figure 15–2.  Decision Tree for Sore Throat Management

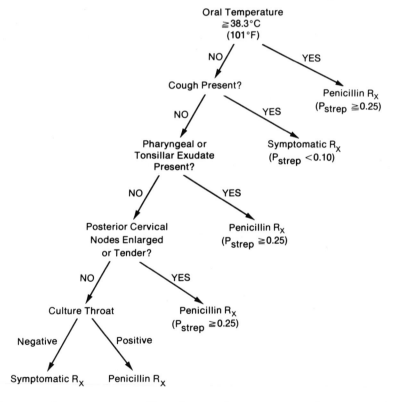

patients, the rate was 4%, about the same as for asymptomatic carriers.

TABLE 15-2.  Comparison of Physician and Algorithm Management of
Pharyngitis

|                          | Antibiotic treatment | |
|--------------------------|-----------------|-----------------|
|                          | Internists      | Algorithm       |
| Positive throat culture  | 85%  (33/39)    | 91%  (29/32)    |
| Negative throat culture  | 26% (129/494)   | 31% (101/331)   |

The treatment data are the most important validation of the algorithm, but we also looked at other parameters including illness outcome, total costs, and patient satisfaction. The algorithm reduced costs significantly—especially when the entire spectrum of upper respiratory illness was considered—without any adverse effects on outcome or satisfaction. Much of the cost reduction came from reducing the use of the throat culture.

OPERATIONAL EVALUATION OF THE URI ALGORITHM

Granted that a URI algorithm could reduce costs without impairing effectiveness in a controlled clinical environment, we decided to see what would happen if the URI algorithm (slightly modified) were introduced into a new setting that had never before used algorithms [7]. To examine the impact of each component of the complete algorithm system (medical logic, checklist, and computer-generated audit/ feedback) on the quality and costs of care, we introduced the components sequentially into a "virgin" primary care clinic at the Seattle Public Health Hospital.

The study was divided into seven periods. Baseline data on the treatment of patients with URI were obtained for eight weeks prior to introduction of the algorithm system. Following this, one of the three components of the system (checklist, logic, computer audit/feedback, in that order) was introduced every ten weeks. During the feedback period, all URI patient encounters were "audited" by special computer programs and written feedback was returned to the provider within 24 hours of each encounter. After the final ten-week period, feedback was discontinued but performance still was monitored for three additional periods of 110 days each. These were referred to as "postfeedback periods."

The results of this study demonstrated that the algorithm system can have beneficial effects on the quality and costs of medical care in a clinic that had never before used this methodology. Specific conclusions were:

- The complete system was required to produce maximum benefit and was cost-effective despite the costs associated with computer audit/feedback.
- In actual use, the providers did not realize all of the cost reductions implicit in the algorithm logic because they did not follow the logic as rigorously as possible.
- The computer audit/feedback had a learning effect on the providers who had been trained adequately in use of the algorithm system. Its removal had a minor effect on these providers' performance.

OBSERVATIONS AND CONCLUSIONS

It is clear that it is possible to develop algorithms for patient-care management that are explicit and reproducible, and that generate quantifiably beneficial effects on the patient care for many common illnesses. These algorithms can be packaged in a cost-effective way that is useful to primary care clinics. The concern that algorithms might cause providers to be insensitive to a patient's hidden problems or to ignore disease not "suspected" by the algorithm has not been borne out by the studies that have examined process and outcome. Algorithms do not produce insensitive robots of caring providers and their use does not compromise relationships with patients [2,7–11].

Additionally, algorithm development has forced clinicians to examine rigorously their approach to clinical management. For instance, it was the attempt to define a cost-effective algorithm for URI that caused us to question the need for throat cultures in all patients with sore throats. This particular test accounted for 31% of the cost of diagnostic tests in patients with URI when it was used routinely for a treatment decision. A cost-benefit analysis resulted from this questioning and a more efficient—but no less effective—approach to managing pharyngitis has resulted.

Obviously, the highly analytic approach used to examine pharyngitis diagnosis and treatment is not necessarily applicable to other illnesses that have been studied less completely or that are more complex. But the same questions need to be asked about the management of other illnesses and, inasmuch as possible, comparisons should be made among alternative, reasonable "algorithms." Although the "best" management of clinical problems may not be defined in this manner, it seems likely that we will learn what is cost effective and begin to define the specific questions that need to be addressed to improve further the decisions that clinicians must make.

It is likely that algorithms will be used more extensively as tools for medical education and standard-setting. They are valuable in this regard, but it is unclear how often they will be used routinely in patient care. Algorithms are most effective in reducing unnecessary use of diagnostic tests, medications, and referrals; but in fee-for-service medicine, there are financial incentives to do more for every patient, regardless of cost effectiveness. It is only in medical care systems where cost effectiveness is rewarded that algorithms have a chance to become more than an academic curiosity.

With regard to management of pharyngitis and prevention of acute rheumatic fever, algorithms can be a useful method to standardize care throughout a community. The algorithms for sore throat evaluations are simple, the data for ongoing evaluation and modification of the algorithm can be collected easily, and new technical advances can be incorporated into the algorithm and evaluated for cost effectiveness. Individual clinics and practitioners can easily monitor themselves for adherence to standards appropriate for their patients and their operational constraints. Only a simple mechanism needs to be established to assist practitioners to develop their own algorithms to collect and use their clinical data, to provide feedback on performance, and to update the algorithms.

## REFERENCES

1. Tompkins, R. K., R. W. Wood, and B. W. Wolcott. 1977. The effectiveness and cost of acute respiratory illness medical care provided by physicians and algorithm-assisted physicians' assistants. *Med Care* 15:991–1003.

2. Wood, R. W., R. K. Tompkins, and B. W. Wolcott. 1980. An efficient strategy for managing acute respiratory illness in adults. *Ann Intern Med* 93:757–63.

3. Tompkins, R. K., D. C. Burnes, and W. E. Cable. 1977. An analysis of the cost-effectiveness of pharyngitis management and acute rheumatic fever prevention. *Ann Intern Med* 86:481.

4. Wood, R. W., P. H. Diehr, B. W. Wolcott, L. Slay, and R. K. Tompkins. 1979. Reproducibility of clinical data and decisions in the management of upper respiratory illnesses: a double-blind comparison of physicians and non-physical providers. *Med Care* 17:767–69.

5. Tompkins, R. K. 1979. Managing pharyngitis

without the throat culture. *J Fam Pract* 8:629–31.

6. Walsh, B. T., W. W. Bookheim, R. C. Johnson, and R. K. Tompkins. 1975. Recognition of streptococcal pharyngitis in adults. *Arch Intern Med* 135:1493.

7. Christensen-Szalanski, J. J. J., P. H. Diehr, R. W. Wood, and R. K. Tompkins. 1982. Phased trial of a proven algorithm at a new primary care clinic. *Am J Public Health* 73:16–21.

8. Charles, G., D. Stimson, M. Maurier, and J. Good. 1974. Physician assistants and clinical algorithms in health care delivery. *Ann Intern Med* 81:733–39.

9. Greenfield, S., F. E. Bragg, D. L. McCraith, and J. Blackburn. 1974. An upper respiratory complaint protocol for physician-extenders. *Arch Intern Med* 133: 294–99.

10. Grimm, R. H., Jr., K. Shimoni, W. R. Harlan, Jr., and E. H. Estates, Jr. 1975. Evaluation of patient-care protocol use by various providers. *New Engl J Med* 292:507–11.

11. Komaroff, A. L., K. Sawyer, M. Flatley, and C. Browne. 1976. Nurse practitioner management of common respiratory and genitourinary infections using protocols. *Nurs Res* 25:84–89.

# 16

# Strategies for Pharyngitis Management: Who Benefits? Who Pays? Who Decides?

*Robert H. Pantell, M.D.,*
*and David A. Bergman, M.D.*

Sore throats bring children and young adults to physicians' offices more often than any other problem [1]. Over 30 million patients are diagnosed each year as having pharyngitis or tonsillitis; at least that number never seek medical attention. Until a decade ago, there appeared to be a consensus among the experts that the optimal strategy for dealing with this problem was to culture symptomatic patients and treat only those positively identified as harboring group A beta-hemolytic streptococci (GABHS). However, there is now considerable disagreement among experts regarding what constitutes sound clinical policy.

Practitioners have their own perspectives, which often diverge from expert recommendations. The record shows that when a diagnosis of pharyngitis is made in a physician's office, nearly 70% of patients do not have their throats cultured, even though 25% receive an injection at the time of the visit [2]. Consensus seems to be universal on only two points: the serious consequences of GABHS pharyngitis (especially acute rheumatic fever) are dramatically declining, and the cost of medical care continues to rise more rapidly than any other item in our economy.

This paper discusses the implications of making certain diagnostic and management choices. The cost analyses that follow are not designed to find a single right answer. Rather they are designed to eliminate choices that are obviously wrong, and to allow us to make rational choices among the remaining explicit alternatives. The use of these decision-analytic techniques will not reduce the uncertainties that are at the heart of the controversies, but will force us to acknowledge the uncertainties and examine the consequences of our decisions at the boundaries of the confidence limits of our knowledge. We shall briefly review the following:

1. The current status of our knowledge about pharyngitis.
2. Create a decision tree to display alternative courses of action.
3. Discuss the concept of utility.
4. Compare the cost effectiveness of proposed strategies.
5. Show how sensitivity analysis can be helpful in judging clinical policies developed with uncertain probabilities.
6. Discuss whether the benefits justify the costs.
7. Suggest how a number of strategies must be utilized rather than a single policy.

## PHARYNGITIS

GABHS infection causes symptoms and suppurative and nonsuppurative complications. All are diminishing in frequency and intensity in a decline that began decades before antibiotics. In the 1980s, it is difficult to determine the precise risk of any of the consequences of GABHS pharyngitis. The best available data are for acute rheumatic fever, but only 36 states report rheumatic fever and reporting of diseases is unreliable. Careful case finding in Baltimore currently reports the incidence rate at 0.5/100,000 [3]. Regional differences are dramatic: California with 10% of the nation's population in recent years has had between 0.6%–3% of reported cases. In 1980, Kentucky had over 20% of the reported cases with less than 2% of our population [4].

The probability that an untreated GABHS patient will develop ARF has only been determined in two studies. An attack rate of 3% was noted in Warren Air Force Base recruits in the 1940s. A penicillin-treated group in the randomized clinical trial experienced a marked reduction in the attack rate to 0.4%. This study is the basis for our current treatment strategy because it demonstrated that ARF can be prevented with penicillin. Ten years later in Chicago, 2/519 untreated children developed ARF (0.4%) compared to 0/532 treated children [6]. Although not statistically significant, the likelihood of a type II error was high. With attack rates of this magnitude, it is unlikely that another randomized control trial will be conducted.

To determine epidemiologically the likelihood of ARF developing following GABHS pharyngitis in the 1980s, we should know precisely the incidence of GABHS pharyngitis, both treated and untreated, as well as the incidence of ARF. While accurate information is unavailable, several studies and surveys will permit us to make an intelligent guess. Studies from the National Ambulatory Medical Survey indicate that each year approximately 11% of school-age children visit office-based physicians for pharyngitis [1,2]. We can estimate therefore that approximately 2% of children will have GABHS pharyngitis. Kaiser reports 8% of children have GABHS pharyngitis per year [7]. Population-based studies in Tecumseh and Rochester indicate that only 12%–25% of sore throats are seen by physicians [8,9]. If we assume that as many as 50% of these have true infections, a 100% medication compliance rate, and a ten-fold reduction in ARF for treated versus untreated cases, we can calculate an attack rate for ARF following GABHS pharyngitis of 1.1–4.5/10,000. As is readily apparent the true attack rate based on these data is dependent upon the assumptions and is somewhat elusive. While we are suggesting an attack rate that has dropped tenfold since the Chicago studies (4/1000) [6], it is important to note that in careful studies the likelihood of developing an ARF recurrence following a documented GABHS infection while receiving prophylactic oral antibiotics has dropped more than tenfold in the past 30 years [10].

The other nonsuppurative complication of GABHS pharyngitis, acute glomerulonephritis, does not seem to be prevented by antibiotic treatment [11]. Suppurative complications have also declined and are currently quite rare. The Warren Air Force Base study of 30 years ago demonstrated that penicillin reduces suppurative complications [12].

Penicillin is effective in shortening the course of scarlet fever. However, despite widespread belief to the contrary, evidence concerning the efficacy of antibiotics in altering the symptomatic course of pharyngitis is contradictory and continues to be debated [13]. No study has compared penicillin with symptomatic regimens. Gargles, cold liquids, aspirin, or acetaminophen may be more effective and safer than penicillin. Therefore, the basis for the antibiotic treatment of GABHS pharyngitis is principally to prevent the development of acute rheumatic fever; preventing suppurative complications is also achievable.

Numerous studies have attempted to identify GABHS pharyngitis on the basis of clinical symptoms and signs.

Certain signs, such as exudate, occur in 70% of GABHS pharyngitis. However, these signs also accompany 65% of viral and 45% of mycoplasmal pharyngitis [14]. Since GABHS pharyngitis currently accounts for only 15% of sore throats, it is far more likely that exudative pharyngitis will have a viral or mycoplasmal etiology. In an era with a low incidence of GABHS pharyngitis, the predictive accuracy of these signs is lower than in the days when 40% of pharyngitis was due to GABHS.

Multiple logistic regression analysis of clinical signs and symptoms has been used recently and has been able to identify a model with 80% sensitivity and 80% specificity [15]. These studies would be aided by looking at antibody titer rises. The standard against which clinical accuracy must be compared is a single throat culture that is capable of detecting 90% of GABHS infections.

In our analysis, it is important to balance the risk of adverse consequences from GABHS infection against the risk of adverse consequences from standard (penicillin) antibiotic treatment. Again a precise figure is elusive, but denominator data are available from military studies and venereal disease clinics. In a study of 27,673 patients without history of penicillin sensitivity, 0.66% experienced a reaction and 0.04% had anaphylaxis [16]. Another study documented one anaphylactic death among 94,655 patients; the military reported no deaths among 315,000 recruits receiving penicillin during a nine-year period [17]. World-wide figures for anaphylaxis are estimated at 0.0015% to 0.004%, with fatalities at 0.0015% to 0.002% [18].

COURSES OF ACTION

When a patient has a sore throat, a number of diagnostic and treatment options are available. Some of the most important are contained in the decision tree (Figure 16-1). In this tree, squares indicate decisions in which there is a choice, while circles represent chance occurrences. The consequences of selecting a particular choice will be discussed shortly.

UTILITY

To judge the effectiveness of a course of action, one must be able to define the expected outcome and to assign a utility to the outcome. Outcomes may be cases of disease detected or prevented, anxiety averted, or increased lon-

Figure 16–1. Sore Throat Decision Tree

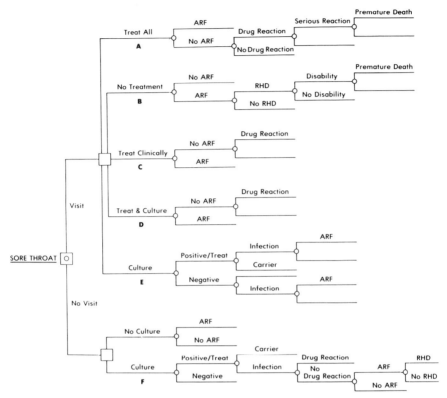

gevity. Utility may be compared on a scale for expressing preferences between outcomes a and b. Frequently, utility is expressed in monetary value. In benefit-cost analysis, all benefits are converted to dollars as are all costs (Tables 16–1 and 16–2). Traditionally, the benefits and costs shown in Tables 16–1 and 16–2 that are indicated with asterisks are not included in such analyses. In cost-effectiveness analysis, a cost is calculated for each case of X detected or (as now fashionable) each quality-adjusted life-year gained [19]. The effectiveness of various strategies can then be compared by looking at the comparative cost for managing Y or giving Z outcome units.

The strengths and weaknesses of these approaches shall soon become apparent. Measuring benefits in monetary terms is fraught with difficulties. While some benefits are easier to calculate (for instance, reduced expenses from avoided hospitalizations), others, such as the cost of life, are more difficult to quantify. The cost of life might be as

TABLE 16-1. Benefits

---

1. Direct
       Saving in medical care costs

2. Indirect
       Increased quality-adjusted life years*
       Increased work capacity and earnings

3. Intangibles
       Increased well-being*
       Decreased pain, anxiety*
       Increased functioning*
       Increased knowledge, satisfaction*

---

*Not included in traditional cost-benefit analyses.

TABLE 16-2. Costs

---

1. Medical care costs
       Direct
           Labor, equipment, materials, medications
       Indirect
           Overhead

2. Patient travel costs

3. Patient opportunity (time) costs
       Lost work*
       Babysitter*

4. Intangible costs
       Inconvenience*
       Anxiety*
       Family functioning*

---

*Not included in traditional cost-benefit analyses.

low as the individual's potential earnings or as high as that person and his social network would be willing to pay to keep that person alive if they all were wealthy. In addition, we must also be aware of the procedure known as discounting health benefits. Since inflation is real, we cannot say that a $90.00 treatment today that brings us a $100 benefit five years from now is a good investment, since an inflation rate of 10% raises the cost of our $90.00 investment to about $145.00. Consequently, if we examined the cost today of a future benefit we usually discount at an annual rate varying from 0%–10%.

## COST-EFFECTIVENESS ANALYSIS

The analysis that follows utilizes certain costs defined in Table 16–3 as well as certain probabilities for events that are defined in Table 16–4. The bases for these probabilities have been discussed and are considered further in references 20 and 21. We use a higher $p$ (ARF/GABHS infection) than we believe is likely, but will alter this probability in the sensitivity analysis section.

Table 16–5 displays the total cost per patient and incidence of ARF using 13 different strategies. It is immediately obvious that strategy D can be eliminated; although its protection against ARF is equal to strategies E, F, and G, it is costlier. The additional cost comes from the increased morbidity of penicillin reactions. Can strategies E and G similarly be eliminated and strategy F be favored? Perhaps. But we know that GABHS pharyngitis is often seen during family stress and may be a family's way of expressing a need to talk with a physician, which may

TABLE 16-3. Cost of Pharyngitis

| | | |
|---|---:|---:|
| Unit costs | | |
| Throat culture | $ | 4 |
| Oral or benzathine penicillin | | 5 |
| Patient time/office visit | | 5 |
| Patient time/pharmacy visit | | 1 |
| Transportation cost/trip | | 2 |
| Initial office visit | | 15 |
| Follow-up visit (injection) | | 5 |
| Daily cost hospitalization | | 120 |
| Adverse outcome costs | | |
| Premature death | | $500,000 |
| Acute rheumatic fever | | 16,734 |
| Serious allergic reaction | | 1,280 |
| Mild allergic reaction | | 26 |

TABLE 16-4. Probabilities: Cost-Effectiveness Analysis

| | |
|---|---|
| p (GABHS/pharyngitis) | .15 |
| p (infection/+culture) | .5 |
| p (+culture/GABHS) | .9 |
| p (ARF/GABHS infection) | .003 |
| p (ARF/treated GABHS infection) | .00034 |
| p (Class IV RHD/ARF) | .039 |
| p (Serious reaction/oral penicillin) | .000083 |
| p (Mild reaction/oral penicillin) | .001732 |
| p ( + clinically/ + GABHS) | .7 |
| p ( - clinically/ - GABHS) | .7 |

reduce the morbidity in such stressful events. This type of potential morbidity cost, as well as many others, is not included in this analysis but must be kept in mind to prevent us from allowing the analysis to dictate rather than to suggest strategies.

When interpreting a table of this type, it is important to look at more than simply the bottom line or total cost. For example, strategy B (no treatment) is cheaper than strategy E (culture and treat). However, the adverse outcome cost for strategy B ($3.77 for ARF cases) is more than four times the cost of strategy E for adverse outcomes (81¢ for ARF and 41¢ for penicillin reactions) when intramuscular penicillin is given. Thus, the net savings of the "non-treatment" strategy B is achieved by decreased patient time and travel and culturing costs but at higher medical morbidity and mortality costs. Trading off reduced patient time and travel costs for higher illness costs is not a decision physicians should make for their patients. The implicit contract between physician and patient is for the physician to minimize the risk of illness.

One might then argue that with this rationale, oral treatment under strategy A has an adverse outcome cost of

59¢ and is preferable to strategies E, F, or G, each with a cost of 83¢. However, this table deals principally with direct and indirect costs and ignores important intangible costs, such as enhancing patient dependence on drug-oriented treatment and promoting the emergence of resistant bacteria. The value of cost-effectiveness analysis rests in motivating the use of alternate strategies when cost differences are large and the number of intangibles and uncertainties is small. A savings of 24 cents does not seem to justify increasing the likelihood of all the above-mentioned intangible costs.

Additional issues for each strategy should be considered:

*Strategy A*: Treat all cases of pharyngitis. This will subject the vast majority of patients to the risks of penicillin allergy. Minimization of false-negative throat cultures is not a major issue when rheumatic fever is so rare.

*Strategy B*: Do not treat patients with pharyngitis. In parts of the United States where rheumatic fever has virtually vanished, the risk of penicillin anaphylaxis may actually exceed the risk of rheumatic fever. In such areas, particularly if the decreasing incidence of rheumatic fever continues, this becomes a reasonable option. If this policy were adopted, it would be important to monitor closely trends in incidence of both ARF and suppurative complications. Although rheumatic fever has been documented in American children less than three years of age, it is so unusual that treatment of pharyngitis in this age group is unwarranted. However, this group may warrant treatment to prevent suppurative complications, an issue not considered here. Certain constellations of symptoms in adults (for instance, cough, absence of fever, and no strep contact) [22] and children [15,7] yield positive culture rates that are not different from asymptomatic carrier rates and support this strategy. Using these symptom clusters may allow us to selectively eliminate this group from culturing or treating.

*Strategy C*: Treat "clinically" suspected pharyngitis patients for ten days. This is the favored approach for patients having symptoms that have a predictivity for streptococcal disease that approaches that of a throat culture. Very few symptom clusters fulfill this criterion (scarlet fever or a combination of petechiae of the palate and moderate redness of the throat), and they comprise only a small percentage of patients with sore throats. This strategy may be resorted to in special situations with patients unlikely to be seen again (for example, migrant farm workers). If suspicion is high that a child may be

TABLE 16-5. Outcome and Cost of Alternative Treatments of 100,000 Patients with Sore Throat

| | A<br>Treat<br>all | B<br>No<br>treatment | C<br>Treat<br>clinically | D<br>Treat orally<br>2 days,<br>await<br>culture | E<br>Culture<br>and<br>treat | F<br>Throat<br>culture only<br>and treat | G<br>Visit<br>optional,<br>culture<br>and treat |
|---|---|---|---|---|---|---|---|
| Acute rheumatic fever (ARF) cases | 2.6 | 22.5 | 9.6 | 4.8 | 4.8 | 4.8 | 4.8 |
| Serious oral penicillin reactions | 8.3 | 0 | 3.0 | 3.4 | 1.2 | 1.2 | 1.2 |
| Mild oral penicillin reactions | 173.2 | 0 | 62.4 | 70.1 | 26.0 | 26.0 | 26.0 |
| Cost/patient treated orally: | | | | | | | |
| Pharyngitis management | $20.00 | $15.00 | $16.83 | $21.02 | $19.75 | $5.50 | $12.63 |
| ARF | .44 | 3.77 | 1.61 | .81 | .81 | .81 | .81 |
| Allergic reaction | .15 | 0 | .05 | .06 | .02 | .02 | .02 |
| Patient time and travel | 10.00 | 7.00 | 8.08 | 8.21 | 7.45 | 7.45 | 7.45 |
| Total | $30.59 | $25.77 | $26.57 | $30.10 | $28.03 | $13.78 | $20.91 |
| Serious intramuscular benzathine penicillin reactions | 213.2 | 0 | 76.8 | -- | 32.0 | 32.0 | 32.0 |
| Mild intramuscular benzathine penicillin reactions | 100.00 | 0 | 36.0 | -- | 15.0 | 15.0 | 15.0 |

212

TABLE 16-5. Continued

| | A Treat all | B No treatment | C Treat clinically | D Treat orally 2 days, await culture | E Culture and treat | F Throat culture only and treat | G Visit optional, culture and treat |
|---|---|---|---|---|---|---|---|
| **Cost/patient treated instramuscularly:** | | | | | | | |
| Pharyngitis management | $20.00 | $15.00 | $16.83 | -- | $20.50 | $5.50 | $13.00 |
| ARF | .44 | 3.77 | 1.61 | -- | .81 | .81 | .81 |
| Allergic reaction | 2.76 | 0 | .99 | -- | .41 | .41 | .41 |
| Patient time and travel | 7.00 | 7.00 | 7.00 | -- | 8.05 | 8.05 | 8.05 |
| Total | $30.20 | $25.77 | $26.43 | -- | $29.77 | $14.77 | $22.27 |

213

developing a peritonsillar abscess or looks particularly toxic, immediate treatment is appropriate.

*Strategy D*: Treat "clinically" suspected pharyngitis patients orally for two days and continue treatment only if the throat culture is positive. This will expose an unnecessary number of patients with viral pharyngitis to the side effects of penicillin without apparent benefit for those with GABHS pharyngitis, since symptomatic relief is probably not enhanced with antibiotic treatment. Furthermore, patients with GABHS pharyngitis and false-negative cultures will not be treated long enough to prevent ARF. This is not a reasonable or cost-effective alternative.

*Strategy E*: Culture all patients with sore throats and treat those with positive cultures within 48 hours. Although more costly overall than some other strategies, this approach minimizes illness and costs associated with illness. Because many patients will be clinically well after 48 hours, explanations of the basis for antibiotic treatment should be given. Withholding antibiotics for up to 48 hours is not synonymous with denying treatment; symptomatic relief for fever and pain can be achieved with either acetominophen or aspirin.

*Strategy F*: Obtain an office throat culture without a physician seeing the patient. Although home throat cultures or office visits for throat cultures alone are effective and economical, GABHS pharyngitis is often seen during family stress and may be associated with a family's need to talk with a physician. Therefore, a policy that eliminates physician visits might reduce the overall quality of care. Allowing patients a choice of visit seems reasonable.

*Strategy G*: Obtain an office or home throat culture; offer patients an optional physician consultation. This is an attractive approach that provides the opportunity to deal with the second "diagnosis." If as many as one-half of patients request a physician consultation, this is still more cost effective than the first five strategies.

BENEFIT-COST ANALYSIS

While cost-effectiveness analysis was used to demonstrate the health resource cost for each case of sore throat managed, we can also use Table 16–5 to examine the cost for each bout of ARF prevented. Strategy G tells us that to prevent 17.7 (22.5 minus 4.8) bouts of ARF, we must be willing to pay 100,000 × ($20.91 minus $0.81) = $2,010,000, or about $114,000 for each case prevented.

Without discounting, we previously assigned a value of $16,734 to the benefit accrued from avoiding ARF. Does this mean that the benefits of treating are considerably less than the costs and that we should discourage treatment? Not necessarily. Remember that the decision to show up at the office is made by the patient. The cost to examine is the marginal cost of preventing rheumatic fever once a patient has incurred the expense of travel and the price of an office visit. For strategy E, the marginal cost for preventing an episode of ARF is $29,440. In this instance, it does not appear that the benefits outweigh the costs. This is not the same as recommending that the strategy be rejected. Consider the long list of benefits we have omitted because of their intangible nature. A lifetime of cardiac anxiety or mild disability can easily be argued to have a cost of more than $100,000. Furthermore, cardiac disability can spell disaster to a professional athlete but have no functional consequences for a computer programmer with a sedentary lifestyle. However, we can conduct a threshold analysis to demonstrate that when GABHS pharyngitis accounts for 25% of sore throats or the ARF attack rate per GABHS pharyngitis increases to 0.005, the benefits do exceed the costs.

Strategy G offers an interesting trade-off. Whereas patients paying for an office visit still have a greater ARF cost than benefit, society on the whole accrues $486,000 when oral penicillin is used: (100,000) × ($25.77 minus $20.91). Parents and children may also accrue additional benefits by being encouraged to participate in the process of medical decision making. Another important consideration is that most patients are risk averse. In other words, empiric studies show that most patients (and doctors) are willing to take more than a mathematically predicted guar- anteed minor loss to avoid the risk of a major loss (that is, they would be willing to pay $50.00 to avoid a 1-in-10 chance of losing $450.00). This tendency to risk aversion probably leads many patients to consider the "monetary" loss in health benefits to be greater than the "monetary" costs of throat culture.


SENSITIVITY ANALYSIS

It has already been established that the confidence interval for some events is extraordinarily wide. In such instances, it is customary to perform a sensitivity analysis in which calculations are performed for varying probabilities within the confidence interval [19]. For example, if the likelihood of developing ARF following a strep throat is as low as 1/100,000 and treating strep throat results in one immediate anaphylactic death for every 100,000 cases treated, it is immediately obvious that no treatment is preferable to treatment. Sensitivity analyses suggest changes in preferred treatment strategies when one probability is altered with all others remaining the same. We shall use sensitivity analysis to demonstrate that the attractiveness of management strategies changes when one alters the probabilities of certain outcomes. In Figure 16–2, we look at four strategies—A (treat all); B (no treatment); E (culture and treat); and F (visit option/culture and treat)—as we vary the likelihood of developing ARF following pharyngitis from

Figure 16–2. Sensitivity Analysis

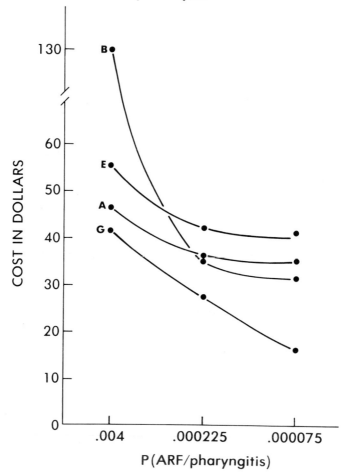

4/1000 to 7.5/100,000. In both Figure 16–2 and Table 16–6, $p$ (ARF/pharyngitis) incorporates both $p$ (GABHS/pharyngitis) and $p$ (ARF/GABHS). Several new costs are used, including cost for an office visit = $25, cost for throat culture = $10, and cost of ARF = $25,000. At $p$ (ARF/pharyngitis) = 0.004, strategy G appears to be the least costly. However, Table 16–7 shows that strategy A prevents an additional 35.4 cases of ARF; the absolute cost for preventing each case of ARF (Table 16–8) for any of the strategies is considerably less than the $25,000 cost we determined as the medical care cost of having a case of ARF. In essence, strategy A offers the best option by permitting 35.4 additional opportunities for saving nearly $12,000 when $p$ (ARF/pharyngitis) = 0.004. At $p$ = 0.000225, we are at approximately the same situation we have previously discussed and the same arguments apply

TABLE 16-6. Cost of Sore Throat Management (in 1983 Captiva Island dollars)

| p (ARF/pharyngitis) | A (treat all) | B (treat none) | E (culture and treat) | G (culture/visit option) |
|---|---|---|---|---|
| .004 | 47.83 | 130.00 | 56.70 | 41.70 |
| .000225 | 36.88 | 35.62 | 42.08 | 27.08 |
| .000075 | 36.33 | 31.87 | 41.33 | 16.33 |

TABLE 16-7. Cases of Acute Rheumatic Fever

| p (ARF/pharyngitis) | A (treat all) | B (treat none) | E (culture and treat) | G (culture/visit option) |
|---|---|---|---|---|
| .004 | 46.4 | 400 | 81.8 | 81.8 |
| .000225 | 2.6 | 22.5 | 4.6 | 4.6 |
| .000075 | .9 | 7.5 | 1.6 | 1.6 |

TABLE 16-8.  Cost Per ARF Case Prevented

| p (ARF/ pharyngitis) | A (treat all) | E (culture and treat) | G (culture/visit option) |
|---|---|---|---|
| .004 | $13,526 | $17,818 | $13,105 |
| .000225 | $185,326 | $235,083 (36,089) | $151,284 |
| .000075 | $550,454 | $700,508 (160,339) | $276,779 |

though the costs are slightly different. However, at $p = 0.000075$, even the marginal cost of preventing a bout of ARF using strategy E is $160,339, a cost that makes one pause and seriously question: Is it worth it? However, strategy G, encouraging patients to selectively request throat cultures, is still considerably cheaper than the posture that, since ARF is so rare, the best thing to do with patients who present to the office is not to culture and not to treat them. It could be argued that at these very low attack rates patients should be discouraged from making office visits for sore throat because it may not be reasonable to spend so much money to avoid a single bout of ARF. However, patients are unlikely to adhere to such a policy. We are left with making the choice of whether to discourage patients from coming to the office when they phone, and whether to culture or treat them when they appear. This type of cost analysis will not tell us at what point to change our policies; it will tell us the cost of a policy. We then must decide if it is worth it.

This sensitivity analysis demonstrates that (1) costs of strategies vary as the probability of acquiring ARF changes, and (2) cost differences for various strategies are often small, signifying that a change in a single cost may reverse ranking. This analysis, used together with benefit-cost calculations, or alternatively expressed as cost per case of ARF prevented, provides us with optimal aid to decision making.

WHO BENEFITS?  WHO PAYS?  WHO DECIDES?

Thus far, this analysis has been conducted in a way that appeals to policymakers. The most cost-effective strategy can be identified, sensitivity analysis has suggested different strategies for different attack rates, and benefits outweigh costs in some instances. However, it is unrealistic to expect that a physician's primary motivation and that a patient's principle concerns coincide with an analytic model that altruistically distributes all benefits and costs equally and demands what is best for society rather than catering to the wishes of individuals. Tables 16–9 and 16–10 list the ranking concerns of physicians and patients. Patients' choices will vary according to factors such as their risk aversion, past illness experience, travel time, and insurance coverage. Physicians, while rendering a service to maintain their patients' health and minimize illness, are also in business and will have preferences that avoid loss of income, medical embarrassment, and malpractice. It is also unlikely that a physician will have the time to perform this analysis (20–30 hours), explain it to each patient (20–40 minutes), and advocate a strategy that will save society costs (no treatment) but allow patients to have a higher rate of ARF than the patients seeing the physician next door. A physician who would jeopardize his income, patients' health, status among peers, and malpractice insurance premium to bow to a societal benefit-cost strategy may be altruistic but is also using questionable judgment.

TABLE 16-9. Doctor Preferences

1. Minimize patient liability
   - disease
   - discomfort
   - disability
   - drug disaster

2. Minimize doctor liability
   - self-esteem
   - malpractice

3. Maximize doctor income
   - dollars
   - resource cost (time)

4. Minimize patient expense
   - dollars
   - time

5. Minimize societal cost

TABLE 16-10. Patient Preferences

---

1. Minimize patient liability
   - discomfort
   - disability
   - disease
   - drug disaster

2. Minimize expense
   - dollars
   - time

3. Minimize societal cost

---

By now, it should be apparent that this type of analysis is useful in that it forces us (1) to be explicit; (2) to define the boundaries of our knowledge, probabilities, and uncertainties; and (3) to examine alternative strategies and trade-offs.

The shortcomings are also plentiful; the analyses are complex and difficult to explain. Physician, patient, and societal preferences may be in conflict. Even the framing of an explanation can evoke differing choices in the same patient. Patients and physicians may not have experience in making choices, given this type of probabilities and risk-gambling criteria.

## WHAT'S A PHYSICIAN TO DO?

Despite the gradual disappearance of ARF in the United States, it is still here. At some point in time, we may wish to say "Stop treating," but this seems neither prudent nor realistic today. Neither physicians nor patients would permit this. The precedent for this type of policy occurred in this country when we discontinued smallpox vaccinations, 25 years after the last case of smallpox in this country. Nevertheless, this strategy may be appropriate in areas with an exceedingly low ARF attack rate. In such areas, office visits for sore throat should not be encouraged, and throat cultures should be reserved for selected situations. In most other areas, patients should be given a choice to decline a physician contact. Office and home culturing are available options.

Some patients who come face-to-face with a physician may be at sufficiently high risk for strep or ARF to merit immediate treatment. These include patients: (1) with past history of ARF; (2) with recent history of ARF in the family; (3) living in an area with an ARF or glomerulonephritis epidemic; (4) with scarlet fever or other constellations of symptoms with high predictivity; and (5) toxic-appearing children. Most patients will have a red pharynx, exudate, or a constellation of symptoms of intermediate predictivity, so that a throat culture should be performed. Up to one-third may have a constellation of symptoms with a high negative predictivity (cough, rhinorrhea, no fever, or strep contact), so that no culture need be taken. Table 16–11 summarizes these recommendations.

TABLE 16-11. Strategies for Managing Sore Throat

| Strategy | Situation |
|---|---|
| | Acceptable |
| 1. Treat all | Epidemic of ARF<br>High-risk patient<br>High p (ARF/pharyngitis) [> .004] |
| 2. Clinical decision | High positive predictivity [> .9]<br>High negative predictivity [> .9] |
| 3. Culture and treat | Standard |
| 4. No treatment | Low-risk patient<br>Low p (ARF/pharyngitis) [> .00001] |
| | Unacceptable |
| 1. Single policy | |
| 2. Treat and culture | |

In the final analysis, physicians must keep abreast of trends in streptococcal illness and local epidemiologic trends. Screening for alloantigens may become practical and may be subjected to cost-effectiveness analysis for comparison to current strategies. In a few years, personal computers will perform cost analyses in a matter of seconds. The utility of this information should be to assist physicians in making choices, rather than making such decisions. If properly used, this can enhance the complex process of physician decision making. It cannot incorporate values or preferences, and, hence, will not replace a good patient-physician interaction for making the ultimate choice.

## REFERENCES

1. National Center for Health Statistics, R. Gagnon, J. DeLozier, and T. McLemore. 1982. The National Ambulatory Medical Care Survey, United States, 1979 Summary. *Vital and Health Statistics,* ser. 13, no. 66. DHHS Pub. No. (PHS) 83–1727. Public Health Service. Washington, D.C.: U.S. Government Printing Office. September.

2. National Center for Health Statistics, B. Cypress. 1979. The National Ambulatory Medical Care Survey, United States, 1975–76. *Vital and Health Statistics,* ser. 13, no. 42. DHEW (PHS) 79–1793. Hyattsville, MD: Public Health Service. July.

3. Gordis, L. This volume.

4. Morbidity and Mortality Weekly Report. 1980. Annual Summary. Center for Disease Control, Atlanta, GA.

5. Denny, F. W., L. W. Wannamaker, W. R. Brink et al. 1950. Prevention of rheumatic fever. *JAMA* 143:151.

6. Siegel, A. C., E. E. Johnson, and E. G. Stollerman. 1961. Controlled studies of streptococcal pharyngitis in a pediatric population. *N Engl J Med* 265:559.

7. Hurtado, A. V., and M. R. Greenlick. 1980. What should be the standard approach to diagnosis and treatment of common, acute respiratory infections and streptococcal sore throats in outpatients? In *Controversies in Therapeutics,* ed. L. Lasagna. Philadelphia: W. B. Saunders.

8. Monto, A. S., and B. M. Ullman. 1974. Acute respiratory illness in an American community, The Tecumseh Study. *JAMA* 227:164.

9. Alpert, J. J., J. Kosa, and R. J. Haggerty. 1967. A month of illness and health care among low income families. *Public Health Reports* 82(8):705–13.

10. Bisno, A. L., I. A. Pearce, and G. H. Stollerman. 1977. Streptococcal infections that fail to cause recurrences

of rheumatic fever. *J Infect Dis* 136:278.

11. Rammelkamp, C. H., C. A. Stetson, R. M. Krause et al. 1959. Epidemic nephritis. *Trans Asso Am Phy* 67:276.

12. Chamovitz, R., C. H. Rammelkamp, Jr., and L. W. Wannamaker. 1960. The effect of tonsillectomy on the incidence of streptococcal respiratory disease and its complications. *Pediatrics* 26:355.

13. Pantell, R. H. 1977. Antibiotics and streptococcal pharyngitis. *Ann Intern Med* 87:632.

14. Glezen, W. P., W. A. Clyde, and R. J. Senior. 1967. Group A streptococcal, mycoplasmas, and viruses associated with acute pharyngitis. *JAMA* 202:455.

15. Williams, T., and R. Lanese. 1982. A Decision Making Model Utilizing a Complex Clinical Data Set. Columbus: Ohio State University College of Medicine.

16. Rudolph, A. H., and E. V. Price. 1973. Penicillin reactions among patients in venereal disease clinics: a national survey. *JAMA* 223:499–501.

17. Frank, P. F., G. H. Stollerman, and L. F. Miller. 1965. Protection of a military population from rheumatic fever. *JAMA* 193:775–83.

18. Idsoe, O., T. Guthe, R. R. Willcox et al. 1968. Nature and extent of penicillin side-reactions with particular reference to fatalities from anaphylactic shock. *Bull WHO* 38:158–88.

# 17

# Management of Pharyngitis

## Discussion

### TREATMENT OF STREP PHARYNGITIS

DR. DENNY: I would like to ask the biostatisticians in the group to comment on compliance and fidelity. It doesn't make any sense to me that if patients have trouble complying with twice-daily medication, it isn't better to administer it four times daily; then if they forget and take medicines twice a day, they're all right.

There is something wrong with the statistics on this, because if you forget just a little bit with twice a day, you should be in a lot worse shape than if you forget a little bit with four times a day.

DR. DILLON: I didn't present any statistical analysis; it's all suggestion.

DR. DENNY: Once-daily medication is obviously not very good, because if you forget a dose you are in trouble.

DR. SANFORD: I'm not a statistician, but I think you have to define what you mean by compliance. A number of studies, particularly in the United Kingdom, have looked at once a day, b.i.d., q.i.d., and two drugs q.i.d. It's clear that the more complex a regimen gets, the less compliant people become. On the other hand, if you are noncompliant with a q.i.d. regimen, you still may get better antibacterial effect than with a b.i.d. regimen. As people write about compliance, they look only at tablet-taking or suspension-taking, not outcome.

DR. SCHWARTZ: In Fairfax County, Virginia, if a child needs a dose during school hours, I have to write on my prescription that the child has permission to keep the medicine at school and that the school nurse can administer the dose. If twice a day is shown to be as effective, it would be much more convenient.

DR. FEINSTEIN: Dr. Denny, I congratulate you for having perceived an increased frequency by improved fidelity, but I'm not sure whether it works where the oral object is a medication!

DR. MARKOWITZ: The recurrence rate or the bacteriologic failure rate has increased perhaps from 10% to 20%, but nothing has happened in terms of purulent or nonpurulent complications. Isn't it as if this bacteriologic failure rate doesn't matter?

DR. DILLON: Well, critical review of many papers over the years reveals that bacteriologic failure rates are not really different. Some of Breese's studies with benzathine penicillin G had failure rates at 30 days, which included perhaps acquisition of new types, in this same 15% to 20% range. But you are absolutely right. I think this is a very important point. That is, with the administration of penicillin as initial therapy, we have seen beneficial effects in terms of the original goals. I think it's only the clinical recurrence that warrants retreatment.

DR. SANFORD: Dr. Dillon, you presented a lot of data on bacteriologic cure and some of the early data on shortening of hospitalization of scarlet fever. One of the arguments between internists and pediatricians is whether treatment of streptococcal pharyngitis shortens the duration of clinical illness. I think we ought to try to decide whether we agree to disagree or whether we agree.

DR. DILLON: Those who will rise to this occasion are those who provided some of the data from the Warren Air Force Base studies. When a recruit was treated on the day of presentation with his illness, differences in duration of fever were observed between treated and untreated individuals. Other things happened, including return of the sedimentation rate to normal more quickly. With scarlet fever, I think the differences were greater. There was also some pediatric evidence along the same line, done earlier. But there has never been a dramatic difference. I don't think anyone would suggest that.

DR. HOUSER: At least in the studies I was involved with, there was a difference between treated and untreated groups at 12 or 24 hours in response of fever. For practical purposes, it was difficult to see much difference in the groups and even more difficult to see for an individual patient.

Now that we are into the age of cost effectiveness, you

might argue that, with even a 12-hour shortening of pain and discomfort and the extra aspirin that would be used without penicillin, it may be cost effective to treat to shorten symptoms.

DR. DENNY: As I remember the data, the patients treated before either 30 or 32 hours of symptoms did show a difference from the untreated group. If treatment was delayed until 48 hours, there was never any difference in symptoms between the treatment and the control groups. As one who made all the double-blind observations in one of those studies, I never could tell which patient was getting medication and which one was not.

DR. STOLLERMAN: I hope somebody will speak of the significance of failure of bacteriologic cure. While we were all impressed with the meaning of that finding to the prevention of rheumatic fever at Warren Air Force Base, most of us who have observed the scene more recently have seen no evidence that those patients who do not achieve bacteriologic cure have a strain that endangers the community—by spreading, leading to rheumatic fever, or infecting secondary contacts. Most of us advise clinicians not to do follow-up cultures, because they are not useful.

During the last decade, the Japanese used enormous amounts of erythromycin for streptococcal infections and produced a population of organisms in Japan that reached 52% resistance to erythromycin, 66% to chloramphenicol, and 90% to tetracycline, at a time when rheumatic fever was disappearing at an astonishing rate in Japan. Those clinicians may have thought they were curing streptococcal disease, but I doubt that they did. I dare say the issue of whether we need bacteriologic cure has to be reexamined in terms of whether the organisms that persist have any relevance to serious infection, rheumatogenicity, and so forth.

DR. AMREN: Clinicians and working parents want to know about communicability of strains. When is the infectious period over? That's perhaps the major reason at this time for treatment after the throat culture is obtained but before the results are available. Perhaps we should discuss when a child can safely go back to school or a day care center after treatment begins.

DR. DILLON: All the data suggest that after 48 hours of penicillin therapy, very few streptococci should be recoverable. Even after 24 hours, the numbers are diminished.

DR. AMREN: Is that also true with erythromycin and cephalosporins?

DR. DILLON: What data there are suggest it's the same

thing. Most people feel comfortable letting a child return to school.

DR. SHULMAN: For the American Heart Association Committee on Rheumatic Fever, I would like to ask if anyone knows of any definitive data regarding prevention of rheumatic fever with cephalosporin therapy of strep pharyngitis.

DR. DILLON: I don't think there are any. And there won't be.

DR. SHULMAN: I wanted to get it on the record.

DR. DENNY: Many people believe that studies done in young adults are not applicable to small children, and yet the few studies that I am aware of strongly suggest exactly the same thing, that the small child is not cured any more rapidly than the adult.

Dr. Schwartz, you said you were convinced that if these patients are treated they get better faster. So is almost every other pediatrician. But do they?

DR. SCHWARTZ: John Nelson and others have data showing definite improvement within a day of treatment. It's almost diagnostic of true infection; if you don't improve within 24 hours of penicillin treatment, even if you had a positive culture, you probably did not have a true infection.

DR. BISNO: Are these controlled studies with a no-treatment group?

DR. SCHWARTZ: Nelson's study had a control group and statistical evidence that symptoms improved very rapidly.

DR. HOUSER: You could do a controlled study by altering your practice of treating immediately and delaying 48 hours for the next group. You would then have an untreated group.

DR. KOMAROFF: Marenstein reported such a study in *JAMA* in the 1970s primarily in adults. He did just what Dr. Houser suggested and found a more rapid resolution of symptoms and signs only in the most toxic subset.

DR. STOLLERMAN: Twelve versus 24 hours.

DR. DENNY: But the Pittsburgh group stated in their study that there was no difference between treated and untreated groups.

DR. PANTELL: In interpreting some of these studies, it's also important to look at the targeted outcomes. Here we are talking about symptoms. No one has yet looked at alternative symptomatic regimens. If we are looking at pain and fever, there are other ways to approach these symptoms, such as with acetaminophen or aspirin. I think some of those studies need to be done.

DR. SANFORD: Dr. Shulman put on the record that

there is no evidence that erythromycin or cephalexin prevents acute rheumatic fever. Is there evidence that penicillin V prevents rheumatic fever?

DR. DENNY: Let's tackle that a bit differently. I believe Dr. Houser showed that failure to prevent rheumatic fever was found in the group that had persistent cultures. Yet, at least a number of the studies done at Warren Air Force Base were done with five days of therapy.

The questions are: What do you need to prevent rheumatic fever, and is the eradication of the streptococcus a marker? I think that needs to really be massaged awhile, because the data still suggest that five days of therapy prevents rheumatic fever in well over 90% of cases.

DR. DILLON: Dr. Stollerman's data in children using penicillin or placebo are the only data I have found in which controlled studies of prevention were done. In the Warren studies, first with oral penicillin and subsequently with intravenous penicillin G, there were gradations in prevention of rheumatic fever. Clearly, a single dose of 600,000 units a day on day 1 was less effective at Warren. The two-dose schedule was a gray zone, and the conclusion was that the three-dose schedule was far better.

DR. STOLLERMAN: Our comparison was with 600,000 and 1.2 million units and we were reluctant to go to 600,000 units every two weeks because we felt it was not as effective as 1.2 million units. We actually had many children whose strep we could not eradicate, something like 12% with 600,000 units. That was still in the days when we felt that the eradication rate was important.

There is one study related to this subject that I always found very interesting. In the early or middle 1940s, Rothbard studied M-typeability and resistance to phagocytosis of strains in the throat during convalescence from streptococcal infection. The investigators found rapid loss of virulence of organisms cultured in the convalescent period with loss of M-typeability and resistance to phagocytosis.

DR. WANNAMAKER: Eradication of streptococci clearly was a mark of success in preventing rheumatic fever. I think all the Warren studies support that.

With attacks rates for rheumatic fever, of course, it's much harder to get a meaningful figure because you don't have very large numerators for calculating attack rates. But I think all the evidence supports the fact that if you really are concerned about preventing rheumatic fever, you had better think about eradicating the organism.

There may be other reasons *not* to eradicate the organism. I think that's the era we are in now. Things have changed, and for some reason we are not seeing rheumatic fever, so maybe it isn't so important to do that. We are treating more carriers now, and I think that's one reason for the high failure rates in our recent studies. I don't think that means that the Warren studies were incorrect.

DR. STOLLERMAN: I didn't say that. I just said we never could figure out what those organisms were doing after they persisted in the throat.

DR. DENNY: I was interested in a comment Dr. Dillon made about prevention of a serologic response. You said that about 12% to 15% of the patients responded with an antistreptolysin-O (ASO) titer.

DR. DILLON: That was in relation to Haight's scarlet fever studies. Other studies show similar suppression.

DR. DENNY: Our data showed that even if treated vigorously with penicillin, virtually 100% of patients develop an ASO response if they are followed long enough. However, if the organism is eradicated, none of them ever develop type-specific antibody.

DR. STOLLERMAN: Yes, type-specific immunity is suppressed very well.

DR. DENNY: But you did not ever completely suppress the ASO response.

DR. STOLLERMAN: We were suppressing primary immune responses in type-specific antibody, while ASO responses are secondary.

DR. DILLON: Some of those papers suggest that ASO responses were indeed suppressed in the treated population at three to five weeks, in comparison to control groups.

DR. DENNY: Yes, and the point I'm making is that you still get a response eventually.

DR. DILLON: The thing that was interesting to me in reviewing those papers again was the fact that you ultimately could separate the suppression of the antibody response, which was originally thought to be important in prevention of rheumatic fever, from eradication, and could show that the latter correlated best with prevention. If I interpret those studies correctly, that was the bottom line. Is that right, Lewis?

DR. WANNAMAKER: Yes, that's correct.

DR. STOLLERMAN: There is another bottom line, and that is the immune response, because in Stetson's data analysis, the magnitude of the antibody response was the best predictor of the attack rate of rheumatic fever in any subset that he analyzed. It could be that there is correlation between eradication of the organism and suppression of the primary antibody response.

DR. DENNY: Yes, but the question is what's important

in rheumatic fever, the primary type-specific response or a different form of response?

DR. STOLLERMAN: That question has never been figured out entirely.

DR. HOUSER: Dr. Gordis, regarding the dramatic change that occurred in the comprehensive health centers that you described, what regimen was recommended in those centers for treatment of streptococcal infection?

DR. GORDIS: They were using penicillin, but the degree of compliance and the proportions of penicillins are not known.

DR. HOUSER: My interpretation of your data was that you attributed the change in incidence of rheumatic fever to treatment in the health centers.

DR. GORDIS: Not on the basis of examining the treatment regimens; on the basis of eligibility and the decline in rheumatic fever preceded by clinical sore throats.

DR. MARKOWITZ: In the clinic population we were in charge of in Baltimore, many of the children were receiving the benzathine penicillin regimen for treatment of streptococcal pharyngitis.

DR. HOUSER: What we have are some studies, now 25 years old, that were carefully done in large populations of young adults. They showed specific things that now either don't apply to children or times have changed. What was established then is irrelevant to the current problem. What I am trying to find out is whether there is other evidence of rheumatic fever prevention in children. Outside of the Baltimore studies of large groups of children, I don't know of any other specific studies that could compare in any way to what was done in young adults.

DR. DAJANI: I would like to bring up the "gold standard" of benzathine penicillin. I asked several people here if they had ever received benzathine penicillin G and most answered no. I have, and it's an exceedingly painful medication. In my mind, that's a definite disadvantage of benzathine penicillin. I'm not sure that, if the pain of pharyngitis versus the pain of the medication is considered, the risk of taking the shot is an advantage.

I still fail to see why any oral cephalosporin should ever be considered for treatment of streptococcal pharyngitis because of the cost and the fact that both oral and gastrointestinal flora are markedly affected by cephalosporins.

DR. EICKHOFF: You are absolutely right about benzathine penicillin. I'm certain that feature of benzathine penicillin plays a major role in the 10% figure for usage, even though we all say that benzathine penicillin is the first-choice therapy for streptococcal pharyngitis. The fact is that it's not being used simply because it is painful. While technically that's not an adverse reaction, it's clearly part of the problem.

With regard to choices of other drugs, I agree with you about the cephalosporins. They are expensive, and clindamycin is expensive. I did not discuss adverse reactions with clindamycin. In one published study, 50 children were given clindamycin for ten days and there was no diarrhea. In another study of 100 children by a different investigator, there was a 25% incidence of diarrhea.

DR. BISNO: On the issue of indications for a cephalosporin, a lot of children have histories, whether true or specious, of penicillin allergy. Our second-line drug is erythromycin, which many pediatricians feel that a number of their patients don't tolerate very well, particularly for a ten-day course. We have told the pediatricians that sulfonamides and tetracyclines are unacceptable, and we really don't make a recommendation for a third-line drug in the patient who is nonanaphylactically sensitive to penicillin and who can't tolerate erythromycin. It seems to me that this is the one rational indication for a cephalosporin.

DR. DAJANI: I will accept that. The only problem is that many physicians are using oral cephalosporins as first choice.

DR. BISNO: No one condones that.

DR. KAPLAN: I would like to inject a word of caution about the recommendations for clindamycin. I have a problem understanding the issues that Brook has pointed out in some of his studies. If clindamycin does what it's purported to do, then so should erythromycin; but the studies that have been presented here, as well as our studies, just don't show the rates of elimination of the "carrier" that he has talked about with clindamycin. Perhaps there are differences between erythromycin and clindamycin I don't understand.

DR. EICKHOFF: I second that comment. In the same paper in which Brook described the eradication of 20 strains of group A streptococci, he also said that a couple of patients with *S. pneumoniae* were not eradicated, so I question the whole thing.

DR. SCHWARTZ: I have a lot of problems with that study. I think there are more than just anaerobes; other organisms can produce beta-lactamase. I just completed a study looking at children who are not in the typical strep age range. Sixteen percent of healthy children six months to three years of age carry beta-lactamase-producing *H. influenzae* in their throats, and somewhat fewer in the nasopharynx. After you give a beta-lactam antibiotic, that jumps to 24% or even higher. Clindamycin, which may be fine for staph and anaerobes, is not particularly good against beta-lactamase-producing *H. influenzae*. I suspect that, in most children, at least up to five or six years, there are more beta-lactamase-producing *H. influenzae* than beta-lactamase-producing anaerobes. In Pittsburgh, for instance, beta-lactamase-producing *Branhamella* is now becoming a major problem in sinusitis and middle ear disease. Clindamycin has been found clinically to be a poor drug against that particular organism. If one is going to examine this, one must look at all beta-lactamase-producing organisms.

DR. SANFORD: As you look through all the compilations you come out with a 10% to 20% failure rate. It's hard to escape the conclusion that eradication must not be the only essential factor in the prevention of acute rheumatic fever. It seems that somewhere there ought to be some rheumatic fever coming through, if you have 10% to 20% failure of eradication.

DR. WANNAMAKER: I think that depends on how you define strep infections. If you have your population of strep infections diluted with a lot of carriers, you are not going to have any risk of rheumatic fever anyway.

DR. SANFORD: I accept that.

DR. TOMPKINS: Regarding the question of why we are not seeing cases of acute rheumatic fever in those instances in which there is a therapeutic failure as measured by the persistence of organisms in the throat, I would like to point out that, even if those organisms there meant that the patient were truly infected, the numbers are so small in an endemic population that you are not going to pick up any cases of acute rheumatic fever in those numbers. I don't think the fact that you don't see them says anything about whether or not the persistence of organisms is important. The numbers are just too small in all those studies.

DR. DENNY: The important thing about Dr. Tompkins' point is that there is still a large group of patients who don't get any treatment who are not getting rheumatic fever right now, so the question becomes almost moot.

DR. EICKHOFF: The majority of the studies that I quoted, and certainly the majority that Dr. Dillon quoted, included patients who were described as having acute pharyngitis. Unquestionably, there are some individuals included who are carriers, because serologic validation was carried out in only a few studies.

DR. FACKLAM: Before we go any further, let me as a microbiologist make a couple of observations. We must interpret some of the failure rates and procedures for documenting the failures of any antibiotic very cautiously. Each of those studies probably used a different technique for isolating streptococci. I suggest that the impression that failure rates have increased over the years is probably due to increased sensitivity of the microbiologic media and techniques.

So if you are using an enrichment or selective-enrichment or selective media, you are going to have a different recovery rates than you would if you were just doing ordinary isolation. When comparing one study to another, you must be very cautious.

DR. DILLON: One reason I chose to present a fair amount of data from Breese's studies was not only that, as Dr. Wannamaker pointed out, his long-term interest and careful observations provide a continuum, but the same bacteriologist did all the bacteriology. That's one reason you see similar patterns there over time. Another point that we don't really talk about in detail is that when we assess "bacteriologic failures," whereas an individual at the onset of infection may have large numbers of streptococci, the recovery of *any* streptococci is often recorded as a bacteriologic failure on return. It's not necessarily an all-or-none phenomenon. If you are concerned primarily about rheumatic fever pathogenesis and the role of the streptococcus, how important is it that the antigenic load of streptococci is quickly diminished, that is getting rid of large numbers of organisms early? When we measure eradication, are we perhaps also measuring the best indicator of getting rid of that antigenic load?

Dr. Dajani and I are in complete agreement about therapy. Some years ago, we practically abandoned intramuscular benzathine penicillin therapy in our clinic population because of a combination of factors. For a lot of children with skin infection, especially younger children, it's a very difficult drug to administer without causing problems. We have achieved satisfactory results in terms of the overall goals of therapy with oral regimens.

DR. WANNAMAKER: Well, I think the question about antigenic load is difficult to answer, but it seems to me that the studies of Cantanzaro and the group at Warren Air Force Base after those of us here had left suggest that if you initiate treatment even as late as nine days, you still prevent most of the rheumatic fever. Even when the antigen load has been there for nine days, you still prevent most of the rheumatic fever. I think that speaks pretty strongly, and it's only one study, against the concept that antigenic load is important.

DR. STOLLERMAN: I have always been impressed with

this issue of antigenic load since, in almost all measurements of rheumatic fever patients' responses to streptococci, the magnitude of the immune response to almost any antigen measured has been greater in rheumatics than in any other streptococcal group. I think that is an important issue.

I have been fascinated by Dr. Wannamaker's allusion to the nine-day delay that still allows prevention. This would be perfectly satisfactory with respect to primary responses. You can prevent primary M-protein type-specific antibody responses up to those nine days. It takes up to 60 days for the specific primary antibody response. Therefore, one of the theoretic considerations has always been, do you really have nine days in which to abort certain immunologic responses? The Warren studies indicate that you do. I think that's an exciting and interesting theoretic issue.

DR. HOUSER: If it is the antigenic load that is important for rheumatic fever and you fail to eradicate the organism, there should be persistence of that antigenic load and risk of rheumatic fever.

DR. STOLLERMAN: No, I don't think so. That's why I mentioned Rothbard and Watson's earlier studies, in that the persisting organisms may bear little relationship in such things as M-protein to the original infection. The rapid changes of these strains that may occur during convalescence may attenuate the organism tremendously.

DR. HOUSER: Is there any evidence that those who have a persistent strain, even though they have been treated with penicillin, develop type-specific antibody?

DR. STOLLERMAN: Those data would be difficult to get. You are asking whether you have better suppression of primary responses in those who are quickly eradicated than in those who have persistence of streptococci. I wish I knew the answer to that.

DR. DENNY: Let me try. Our numbers are relatively small, but eradication by penicillin was so complete that only about one of 20 patients had a positive culture after initial treatment. There was no development of type-specific antibody in that group.

On the other hand, with patients treated with either tetracycline or aureomycin, the recurrence rate was quite high, and a lot of those patients developed type-specific antibody. That is as close as we could come.

DR. DILLON: Does type-specific antibody prevent localized acute streptococcal pharyngitis by the homologous type?

DR. STOLLERMAN: The group at Warren Air Force Base with Siegal looked at type-specific antibody. Lewis, you probably can speak to this best as protection against streptococcal infection. Those people who had type-specific antibodies were protected against natural challenge in the conditions of the experiment. Is that right, Lewis?

DR. WANNAMAKER: Yes, I think the studies clearly showed that the acquisition of a new type that persisted in the throat and in some cases caused clinical disease was correlated with the absence of type-specific antibody and not antibody to other types.

On the other hand, quite a few transitory acquisitions occurred in those individuals who acquired a type to which they had type-specific antibody. They kept the organism only one or two days, and we did not call those infections. I think the more recent studies in Egypt also confirm that it is possible to get these transitory acquisitions whether or not type-specific antibody is present.

DR. BISNO: We on the American Heart Association committee have had much interest from pharmaceutical sources regarding Bass' data on the combinations of procaine and benzathine penicillin. Of course, these have been around for a long time. Are there any data that indicate the procaine mixture really is less painful? I know such data are difficult to acquire, but does anyone have anecdotal evidence from his own gluteus or other data?

DR. MARKOWITZ: I think it makes a big difference, and I think Bass comments on that. We used the combination of benzathine and procaine penicillin in practice for many years, and it was tolerated quite well, in contrast to pure benzathine penicillin G. I don't think there is any doubt that the combination does relieve pain considerably.

DR. PANTELL: There are some trade-offs when you give procaine. I also had some problems with Bass' study in that he had four treatment groups, including one group given 600,000 units of benzathine penicillin. He found a high failure rate in that group, but it included many adults who ordinarily should have received 1.2 million units. Similarly, in his group treated with 1.2 million units of benzathine penicillin, he had many children who should have received 600,000 units, and he found a lot of pain in that group. He really wasn't treating according to current recommendations, giving larger doses to some small children and smaller doses to some adults. This may partially explain the failure rate and also the pain reaction rate.

Another thing that wasn't brought up in the study is the procaine hypersensitivity syndrome. Procaine is not an inert substance, but causes reactions, including tachycardia and extreme anxiety. Before we leap to giving procaine when we give benzathine, we need to consider these trade-offs.

DR. EICKHOFF: The people who use a lot of benzathine penicillin these days are the venereologists. In our clinic in Denver, we don't see much trouble with benzathine penicillin, but we see more problems from the procaine component than we do from anaphylaxis to penicillin.

DR. FERRIERI: Regarding bacterial persistence, I think the issue of penicillin tolerance is interesting and I wonder if anyone else has any solid data to support a possible role of tolerance for group A strep?

DR. GERBER: I don't have any solid data, but I have a word of caution about interpreting the data presented in the study by Sprunt. That study showed a high prevalence of tolerance in the group A strep they examined. As I recall, the organisms were all in the stationary phase of growth. Kim and Anthony, looking at group B strep, have shown that organisms in the stationary phase frequently show a discrepancy between the minimal inhibitory concentration (MIC) and the minimal bactericidal concentration (MBC), which is no longer present when you look at the same organisms in logarithmic phase. I don't think anyone knows the true prevalence and significance of penicillin tolerance in group A strep.

DR. KAPLAN: Kim has looked at about 100 strains of strep that we have sent him from some of our treatment failures. The preliminary evidence suggests three or four strains that may be tolerant.

DR. ANTHONY: By several parameters, they really do seem to be tolerant. He has not looked at autolysis, which is, for instance, the way Tomasz has defined tolerance, but they seem to be tolerant.


## STREPTOCOCCAL CARRIERS

DR. WATANAKUNAKORN: Dr. Kaplan, for clarification, did you classify your group with high initial antibody levels as postinfectious carriers or as contact carriers?

DR. KAPLAN: I think they probably are postinfectious carriers, if you believe that term. In other words, these are individuals who have had an undetected streptococcal infection in the past and have continued to harbor the organism.

DR. WATANAKUNAKORN: How about the contact carriers?

DR. KAPLAN: That term was coined by Kuttner and Krumweide. Many would equate that group with what I prefer to call transient carriers, with very transient acquisition and loss of the organism from the upper respiratory tract.

DR. WATANAKUNAKORN: Would that group have low antibody levels?

DR. KAPLAN: They probably would have low antibody levels and experience no rise in titer because they don't recognize the organism.

DR. TOMPKINS: You used data from Dr. Stollerman's original Chicago study as evidence that the patients with acute rheumatic fever correlate with some other signs of infection. I would like to suggest caution about making too much of that. There were only two patients with acute rheumatic fever in that study. I think the chance of segregating those randomly into some of those subpopulations might lead one to wonder whether that information can be used as solid evidence that infection and acute rheumatic fever correlated.

If you had more than two cases and the denominator were substantially larger, you would be on safer ground, but I'm a little concerned about the numbers there.

DR. KAPLAN: Certainly it is a small number, and one has to interpret it with caution.

I think you are asking for a study that doesn't exist. What you would like is 400 cases of rheumatic fever and 12,000 cases of sore throat. I am sure that I would have to get at the back of the line to volunteer to do such a study if you could find us the population to do it in. At this time, I think we have to go with these data.

DR. TOMPKINS: I'm just cautioning against extending the data too far with those numbers. I think your conclusions are correct. I think your other data are much more convincing.

DR. FEINSTEIN: Dr. Tompkins is referring to what statisticians call a type II error; that is, you conclude that there is no difference when in fact there may be one. It's the risk you take when the numbers are relatively small. In this situation, as Dr. Kaplan pointed out, if you could get better numbers to work with, there would be better numbers. But what I think is remarkable in those data is that the numbers were as large as they were, considering the problems, and I think that's a reasonably remarkable set of information.

I have a question relating to the issue of the carriers having a higher antibody titer when you first meet them in contrast to the other folks. That's a little jarring intellectually because I am thinking of all the house staff who, when patients are admitted to the hospital and they are trying to indict a strep in the background of whatever ailment these folks have, will regularly get a single streptococcal antibody titer. If it's high, they then say, "Aha." It has taken some of us quite a while to educate them to the fact that you ought to get at least a second antibody titer later before you can say no. But it is the "Aha" elicited by that high antibody titer that is somewhat distressing, because your "Aha" is one that says it may indicate carriage when other people are "Aha"-ing in the direction that this demonstrates there was indeed a recent infection.

DR. KAPLAN: I think your comment is correct. We would have said "Aha" the other way a couple of years ago, before these data started to fall out. We caution people about this, and I think it's part of our education not only for our house staff but also for primary care physicians who call with ASO titers of 400 or 600.

DR. FEINSTEIN: Another question arises from guilt harbored for many years by all of us current or former streptococcologists about the way we identify infections. Our avidity of examination of all the antibody titers and the frequency with which we follow patients for those titers are triggered by some event—a clinical ailment, a throat culture, a manifestation of rheumatic fever, nephritis, or what have you. If in response to that event, we then get appropriate changes in the antibodies, we say, yes, we have identified an infection in contrast to a carrier state.

However, as far as I know, there have been no studies in which the same panoply of avid detection procedures have been used in response to other events. If somebody has some other kind of clinical manifestation, we really don't know how frequently we would get these rises, for example, in association with pneumonia, urinary tract symptoms, or other ailments. We don't know how frequently such changes in titers occur in the rest of the population about whom we harbor no suspicion of streptococcal infection.

I find that troublesome because I don't know to what extent a certain amount of these antibody changes may occur in the rest of the world. We have not identified a completely adequate control group for the decisions that we are making about the particular events on which we focus.

DR. KAPLAN: The point is well taken and it's hard to respond to, except to point out that, in the study I quoted, there were 113 asymptomatic individuals with negative cultures who were index patients, and we found about a 5% rise in titer. I have always felt good about that 5% because if it had been 0%, nobody would have believed the studies.

DR. TARANTA: With regard to the "Aha" controversy, it depends on the time at which one makes the determination. That is, if one makes the determination of an ASO titer when the patient comes into the hospital with acute polyarthritis, it is one thing. If one makes the determination when the patient comes into the emergency room with an acute sore throat, it is another thing. In the first instance, a high ASO titer is indicative of a previous infection and, therefore, will tilt the balance in favor of a diagnosis or possible complication. In the second case, a high titer cannot be due to that particular infection because the infection has lasted only a day or two. Therefore, this tilts the balance, if the throat culture is positive, in favor of a carrier state.

Concerning the other point, Dr. Feinstein and I were associated in running a clinic in which we performed routine ASO examinations, so at least we are intimately acquainted with a population of some 500 children in whom we did ASO titers regardless of findings. In fact, we did such determinations in the presence of a number of intercurrent infections that were known not to be streptococcal related, and no ASO rise was usually associated with such events.

DR. FEINSTEIN: But in that clinic, when the antibody titer rose and there had been no corresponding set of clinical manifestations that fit our preconceptions, we said "Aha, there has been an intercurrent streptococcal infection."

DR. TARANTA: But we had a number of patients with other diseases, such as juvenile arthritis, pneumonia, and so on, and no increases in titers were found.

DR. DENNY: Dr. Kaplan, you said that a carrier is one who does not develop an antibody response. But that does not mean that that person did not develop that carriage following an earlier infection. So it is just a question of timing. The question I have is whether a patient ever contracts a streptococcal carriage state that continues for weeks or months without ever being infected with that organism. That is the critical issue that we are talking about. Otherwise, your definition of a carrier seems rather wishy-washy.

DR. KAPLAN: No, it's time related. It doesn't make any difference, at least from the point of view of prospectively dealing with that individual, what happened earlier, because if he or she were to develop rheumatic fever, as we have discussed here, the period of risk probably was sometime in the past. What I am concerned about from the point of view of the practitioner is what happens from here to there.

In answer to your question, the literature describes patients with prolonged "carriage," or harboring, or colonization, or whatever term you choose, who have been followed by a number of parameters and who continue to harbor the organism with falling or level antibody titers over a prolonged period.

DR. DENNY: Were they observed to go from a culture-negative state to a culture-positive carrier state without an antibody response?

DR. KAPLAN: You can answer that question by pulling together several studies that include patients who have gone from the negative state to a positive state and then have lost it again. You can also find studies of individuals who, from the time they are identified as having the organism, show falling titers. I can show you numerous examples of this, but I have no way of telling how common it is.

DR. WANNAMAKER: We have some information that will help to answer several of these points. Some data from the Warren Air Force Base studies and some more recent data of Dr. Ayoub's clearly indicated that you can have a carrier state without developing antibodies. How common, it is hard to say. One problem in interpreting these data is that there are quite a few "spotty carriers," so if you have a negative culture you are not sure whether it's a new acquisition the next time the patient is cultured and is positive. You have to have a whole series of negatives, I think, and even then you may not be entirely sure that it's a new acquisition, because frequently these carriers are carrying small numbers of organisms and it's a sampling problem.

In answer to Dr. Feinstein's question, I think there is clear evidence that you do not get changes in antibody without finding a streptococcus. There have been studies, including the one at Warren, that correlate acquisition and persistence of the organism with the development of antibodies. This has been done more recently in Egypt, where not all had group A—some had Cs and Gs—but I think as far as ASO is concerned, you can explain that by the fact that these non-group As do produce this response.

DR. BISNO: Dr. Kaplan, there are data to indicate that in individuals who have high initial titers, it's more difficult to demonstrate a rise in antibody titer. Ranz showed this for pharyngeal infection, and we showed it for cutaneous infection. In previous studies, you have answered that criticism by looking at the opposite antibody and showing that it would go up. In your data here, you had both high mean ASO and anti-DNase B titers in this group of patients. Can you rule out that at least some of your results are because those people were less able to mount a demonstrable immune response because of their high initial titers?

DR. KAPLAN: Is your question whether this group is different from the group we reported about ten years ago?

DR. BISNO: In the earlier group, you showed that the other titer was low and then rose. But in this group, your mean titers are high for both ASO and anti-DNase B.

DR. KAPLAN: I have not analyzed these data as thoroughly as I did those ten years ago. I don't have a complete analysis of that. I think it seems unlikely, but it's possible.

DR. BISNO: I also want to ask about your failure rates with benzathine penicillin, which are in the range of 19% to 28%. It's clear that your selection of patients was different from the usual selection. Most studies are based on people walking into a pediatrician's office, whereas yours were based on identifying index cases and their family contacts and on using nasal and salivary cultures as well as throat cultures. Do you think your 28% failure rate indicates some difference in the ecology of streptococcal disease, or is it purely due to differences in the selection of the patient population?

DR. KAPLAN: It's hard to know how to take all factors into consideration. The first study was in an outbreak situation in a semiclosed community in St. Paul, Minnesota. The second study, which I just reported, was in an endemic situation and included individuals going to a hospital ambulatory clinic.

DR. BISNO: Even in the outbreak, didn't you extend your studies into families and do multiple cultures from multiple sites?

DR. KAPLAN: Not in the outbreak studies.

DR. GERBER: Some people feel that not only is treatment of carriers not indicated in order to prevent spread or nonsuppurative sequelae but actually may be contraindicated because that is the manner in which we develop antibodies to strep. Are there data to support those claims? Is the carrier state beneficial?

DR. SHULMAN: To drug companies or to patients?

DR. KAPLAN: In theory, I think you are right; but I'm not sure that studies have been done.

DR. MARKOWITZ: I think Dunlap and Harvey showed that, using the long-chain technique.

DR. HOUSER: Back in the days when it was important to culture and treat positive cultures, one of the problems with chronic carriers was that they were cultured every time they came in with a respiratory infection; the culture would be positive, and they would be treated. At least one indication for trying to eradicate the chronic carrier state was to prevent the misdiagnosis every time the child came in with a positive culture. It may not be germane any more.

DR. SCHWARTZ: All these studies are based on tests that may be antiquated in the next few years, the ASO titer and the anti-DNase B titer. With more sophisticated techniques, such as using monoclonal antibodies, these data might be very different.

Did you look at those with rapid falls in titers that might have been indicative of something like a smoldering infection wtih a rapid flare-up of symptoms, a high titer at that point, and a rapid fall over the next month or six weeks? I wonder if you should consider that as an active infection also.

DR. KAPLAN: We have looked at that and it doesn't change our data particularly. In response to your first comment, I'm not quite prepared, despite what the monoclonal people can do, to conclude that the ASO and the anti-DNase B will be antiquated very soon.

DR. FEINSTEIN: I want to respond to a question asked by Dr. Denny. It seems to me that Dr. Kaplan's carriers for whom the geometric mean is evaluated are a mixture of noninfected people who probably have low antibody titers, plus another group who might be called slow decayers who had an infection previously with an antibody response that has taken a long time to go down. Thus, when we encounter them, they have an elevated antibody titer, and that group—I think you called them postinfectious carriers—is mixed in with the noninfected group to form this carrier group, and you then find that elevated geometric mean. My guess is there are two populations in there.

DR. KAPLAN: You are suggesting that the responses would have a bimodal distribution. I don't think we have found that.

DR. FEINSTEIN: The mere fact that the data didn't fit the speculation should not stop you.

DR. DENNY: They never have. Why stop now?

DR. TARANTA: The definition of *carrier* depends largely on our technical ability to detect antibodies. In an extreme case, if only the ASO titer is determined, one would then misclassify as carriers a number of patients who have active infection. The more antibody titers you do and the more accurate they are, the fewer the number of carriers and the greater the number of infections.

It might be interesting to try another method in the

study of carriers, such as the ratio of actively dividing cells to total cells. Maybe this is becoming possible.

DR. KAPLAN: There is a technique for that and we intend to start looking at this.

DR. STOLLERMAN: Before we leave the review of the studies at Children's Memorial Hospital, I would like to remind you that there were almost 300 cases in our untreated group of patients in whom we clearly showed a titer rise of antibodies, including ASO, and no cases of rheumatic fever.

I make this point so that you don't dismiss the lack of rheumatic fever entirely on the basis of the carrier issue. We were seeing the kind of streptococcal infection that others have also seen, in which there are antibody rises when you measure these very sensitive tests (and I would say that the ASO is a supersensitive test) in which there is no rheumatic fever. Therefore, my interpretation has been that that is a different kind of infection, either quantitatively or qualitatively, with regard to the attack rate of rheumatic fever.

But I still say that all the data should come out. In Dr. Bisno's studies, even rheumatic fever may not recur where there are confirmed antibody rises in rheumatic subjects. We don't have enough good prospective data to confirm that all the antibody rises were due to a group A strep. Undoubtedly, some of Dr. Bisno's data may have been due to rises due to streptococcal groups G, C, and others.

But even in the rheumatic population, individuals with antibody rises these days do not have the same rate of recurrences of rheumatic fever that we saw ten and 20 years ago.

DR. KAPLAN: Your point is well taken. There are two ends to this axis, if you will, one being the host and the other the bacterium.

DR. STOLLERMAN: I'm emphasizing the bacterium, because that's one I can look at.

DR. DENNY: But let's bring in chance again on this. In Wyoming, there were times that we saw several hundred group A streptococcal infections without any rheumatic fever, only to find the next hundred infections associated with ten cases. Everything indicated then, and I believe suggests even now, that this is a chance phenomenon.

DR. HOUSER: That has always concerned me, too. What was the evidence in the population that your patients came from that rheumatic fever was or was not occurring? Siegel said there had been cases in siblings of these children and that this was something he really didn't know how to handle.

DR. STOLLERMAN: As far as I know, there was a spectacular decline in the rate of rheumatic fever in that population that occurred over five to ten years. The rheumatic fever ward of 40 beds at Children's Memorial Hospital eventually closed.

## DECISION ANALYSIS AND ALGORITHMS

DR. HOUSER: Dr. Pantell, you suggested that treating or waiting on the results of the throat cultures were both strategies. One problem is that you are looking at cost spread over a population.

It seems to me that you have to consider also the epidemiology, if you will, of streptococcal infections in the population. We have heard nothing here to suggest that the mechanism of transmission of streptococcal infections has changed. It seems to me that you have to include in such a model the risk of that two days of untreated streptococcal infection in transmission, creating other cases in the community, because you are looking at the impact on the total community. Would it change your strategy or your outcome to include additional cases that resulted from not treating these children for two days?

DR. PANTELL: This is one of the almost limitless number of things that we can factor into a cost analysis, and it's also one reason I am usually reluctant to perform this type of analysis. This certainly could have a dollar value factored in. However, it seems to me that the way throat cultures are used by physicians in the community, if we accept the figures presented earlier in this meeting, is what I am concerned about as much as the type of physician who exposes patients to adverse reactions.

I can't tell you right now if the risks of penicillin are any greater in those patients than the risk of transmission to other individuals.

DR. HOUSER: Perhaps we should look only at the behavior of the disease as it is in patients who present, without taking into consideration the behavior of the disease in the population, and the way these strategies may impact on that.

DR. FORSYTH: Dr. Tompkins, can you give us any estimate of the cost of developing and maintaining algorithms? Algorithms are not stable and require a lot of maintenance, such as introducing new information from the literature and epidemiologic information. I think those costs were not represented in your cost analysis.

DR. TOMPKINS: I don't know the costs of developing

the original ones because a lot of work went into them. But it is clear that we are a long way from the beginning now and, at least for sore throat management, most of the algorithms that have been developed in different places are beginning to look similar.

There are some differences between populations, especially between children and adults. But my guess is that right now, if this group were to specify the parameters that it thought were most useful in differentiating patients with positive and negative cultures, we could go back to data from several populations to construct an algorithm and give you an indication of how well it worked.

The bigger job is to make sure the algorithms work the way they are supposed to work. I don't think you need to do a lot of tests. I estimate that, if an algorithm were used, data collected, and the same kind of follow-up done as if we were not validating an algorithm, evaluation of 300 to 400 patients will tell you whether the algorithm is working the way you want it to work. After that you can spot-check it regularly, so that the cost is relatively small.

Most algorithms are safe for most practices, and you can maintain quality control as you go. I don't think they change so much epidemiologically as they do in terms of the way in which the practice must operate.

DR. BISNO: I wonder if the algorithm approach being used now is directed at the right thing, since most algorithms are understandably focused upon the most cost-effective way to prevent rheumatic fever.

I wonder if the questions we face right now in the community aren't different questions entirely. As we have heard in this conference, rheumatic fever is declining dramatically. We don't have the foggiest idea of how much of that decline is due to factors related to the organism, factors related to the environment, or factors related to the host, and indeed how much of it is due to what we have called primary prevention.

There is some question now, when the incidence of rheumatic fever is so low, regarding just how effective the classic and traditional primary prevention of rheumatic fever really can be.

In this setting, it seems to me that we face another issue: Given that we are not ready to abandon all treatment of sore throat because of the chagrin factor or the adverse risk factor, it seems that we have a real obligation to minimize the amount of antibiotic that we use in treating a lot of patients with sore throat who have an extremely low risk of rheumatic fever.

Any strategy we look at nowadays has to be examined

very seriously from the standpoint of how much *treatment* it prevents, perhaps as much as if not more than how much *rheumatic fever* it prevents. Dr. Tompkins, are there algorithm strategies that minimize the amount of treatment to the same extent that a negative throat culture does?

DR. TOMPKINS: One of my figures showed a comparison between internists using the traditional culture-and-treat technique and those using an algorithm. A little more antibiotic was given with the algorithm, but the difference between the two groups was barely significant.

DR. BISNO: Was that because the internists didn't do things the way they should have done them?

DR. TOMPKINS: Their behavior mimicked behavior in other parts of the world. There are numerous reasons that people get antibiotics unnecessarily. A variety of other pressures may apply. Regardless of whether the algorithm could work better or doesn't work better, it worked as well as at least one group of physicians, and there is some comparison with others.

I would like to address the issue about what an algorithm is supposed to do. These were designed to try to predict patients without having to obtain a throat culture. A major concern in some algorithms was reducing costs to the institution and costs to the patient. Particularly the algorithm that attempted to keep patients from having to come in to see a provider was designed to do that.

Another motivation was to try to get treatment to people as early as possible; for all the reasons discussed here, there are major advantages in treating potentially positive strep patients early. A third motivation was to prevent doing much to those people who aren't likely to have anything done to them, who are in the majority; they would not have a throat culture done, with its expenses, nor would they be given penicillin. The rheumatic fever analysis I did for the decision analysis was designed to give me some parameters, given that that was a major reason for treating patients with strep pharyngitis.

DR. FEINSTEIN: I want to reassure Dr. Tompkins and Dr. Pantell that I know that flow charts can be used to show the logic and the reasoning, but they were not designed that way. In the usual computer model or pathway it's not there, and if you want to put it in, you have to arrange for bells, buttons, whistles, and so forth, and be able to show what the reasoning was.

DR. KOMAROFF: Is there a subset of patients in whom, based on clinical findings, the risk of strep is so low that you would advocate eliminating the throat culture?

DR. TOMPKINS: Absolutely.

DR. KOMAROFF: Who are they?

DR. TOMPKINS: About half the patients—those who don't have fever, who don't have an exudate, who usually have a cough, perhaps who are over the age of 35—are in a low-risk group. Most of them don't need to have anything done.

DR. KOMAROFF: The reason they don't is not just to save money of the throat culture but also the risk that the culture will be false-positive and that treatment will be unnecessarily given and that unnecessary morbidity will be created in some patients? Are you making the recommendation based not only on saving immediate dollars but also on a risk-benefit balance?

DR. TOMPKINS: It's based on the decision-analysis work that suggests that it doesn't make much sense to treat those low-risk populations. In addition, the throat culture rates in those populations are basically the same as you find if you culture the population randomly, so they probably are carrier groups.

DR. BISNO: Isn't there general agreement on that without algorithms? I think everybody would agree that an afebrile 35-year-old man without any exudate doesn't need a throat culture.

DR. TOMPKINS: It's remarkable how many people are treated.

DR. HOUSER: We are talking as though there is an algorithm reflex to the guidelines that were set up to recognize and manage streptococcal infections. I don't think it has ever been the intent to eliminate physician judgment. If physicians cannot judge whether or not to get a culture and have to depend on an algorithm, there is something wrong with the way we have trained them. That's why I don't understand how you can identify people who shouldn't have a throat culture.

DR. TOMPKINS: Dr. Houser, the algorithm that everybody who shows up with a sore throat gets cultured is what we have used previously.

DR. HOUSER: That's my point. It has been interpreted as an algorithm, but I don't think the intent was ever that it should be an algorithm.

DR. TOMPKINS: An algorithm is merely a set of rules, and that's a rule.

DR. HOUSER: If physicians want to interpret that as a rule, then they are doing away with their right to make judgments and to understand the natural history of streptococcal infections, respiratory infections, and so forth, and to use judgment that presumably we have been trying to put into them.

DR. FEINSTEIN: The problem is that, magnificent though it is, our medical education often does not produce the kind of judgment you are assuming it does. Part of the reason is that our splendid faculty will often not specify the ingredients of what they are thinking about and the way they are thinking about it and produce that in a specific, transmissible way so the recipients of that information can begin to make use of it and incorporate it into their own judgment. Very often we get faculty members who say the reason to do something is that it works, or that it gave terrific results in the last 500 rats in the laboratory, or that there is a splendid pathophysiologic rationale, like giving high-concentration oxygen to premature infants. Those reasons don't produce terribly good clinical judgment.

It seems to me the great virtue of the algorithm makers when they try to go through this sort of thing is not necessarily the quantitative results that emerge, but, first, the realization that they impose on all of us that the information we need isn't there and that as investigators we have failed to get it and make it clear; and, second, that it imposes upon us as teachers the need to recognize what goes into these judgments, how we think about them, and how we specify them.

I think for both of those reasons the approach is an excellent one. My quarrel is really with the numbers that are thrown in, not with the approach.

DR. DURACK: Dr. Feinstein, you gave us an eloquent explanation of what a strong force the chagrin factor could be. My problem is that this varies tremendously among physicians, unlike the cost of a throat culture; and physicians vary enormously. For example, residents are much more chagrined by leaving a patient untreated overnight than an attending physician would be. Doesn't that invalidate a lot of the decision analysis?

DR. FEINSTEIN: I was neither trying to invalidate the analysis nor trying to validate it; I was simply trying to indicate how it gets done. I think that the chagrin factor changes at different stages in life. As a resident stops worrying that somebody is going to reprimand him in the morning for not getting that full workup, he may then discover it is possible not to get the full workup that night and not be chagrined.

I think the decision as to what makes chagrin will vary from one physician to another and from one patient to another. In circumstances where patients increasingly are being invited to join in decision making, and are beginning to demand to join in that decision making, recognition of what produces or might produce chagrin for the patient, the physician, or both is what gets involved when a lot of these decisions are being made.

I didn't say it leads to a correct or an incorrect decision; I am simply saying that if you look at the factors that lead to the decision, chagrin is important.

DR. FORSYTH: One problem is that some of the recommendations involve electing not to obtain data. Of course, the driving force in much of medicine is always to acquire data, and to acquire more and more certainty. The intolerance of uncertainty is a variant of the chagrin factor, and most students and residents are taught to reduce uncertainty by acquiring more data.

# 18

# Management of Pharyngitis in an Era of Declining Incidence of Rheumatic Fever: An Overview and Synthesis

*Jay P. Sanford*

The central theme about which the conference has been designed is, "How does or should the medical profession respond in an appropriate manner to the apparent disappearance of a disease?" From the historical perspective, there are a number of infectious diseases that have either been eradicated or whose prevalence in the United States has become extremely low. With the eradication of smallpox, immunization with vaccinia has been discontinued except for laboratory personnel who are working with vaccinia and for active duty military, where there is concern about smallpox as a biological weapon. With control of typhoid primarily through sanitation and other public health measures, immunization against typhoid is no longer recommended. In contrast, while the number of cases of naturally acquired paralytic poliomyelitis has been less than ten per year over the past decade, its occurrence in pockets of nonimmune individuals provides a sound basis for the need for continuing immunization. Similarly, while the incidence of tetanus has declined markedly, this is due to a major extent to ongoing programs of active and possibly passive immunization. Dr. Gordis presented data that suggested that the decrease in acute rheumatic fever may be related to the provision of medical care to symptomatic individuals; however, to draw analogies between smallpox or poliomyelitis and acute rheumatic fever is difficult, because it is not certain why the incidence of acute rheumatic fever has decreased.

There is general consensus that the primary purpose for the diagnosis and treatment of group A streptococcal pharyngitis has been the prevention of acute rheumatic fever. Before concluding that recommendations should be drastically modified, it is important to consider other reasons why diagnosis and antimicrobial therapy may be indicated. First, treatment may result in the more rapid alleviation of symptoms. Unfortunately, although most physicians and patients believe that penicillin treatment shortens the duration of the acute illness, Dr. Denny pointed out that, if treatment was begun before 30 to 32 hours of the onset of symptoms, there was a shortening of illness that was not observed if the delay was 48 hours. As an observer in a double-blind study, he (Dr. Denny) was unable to distinguish between penicillin and nontreatment. Second, treatment may prevent or decrease the likelihood of suppurative complications. This aspect was not discussed, although most participants would probably agree with the statement.

Allow me to reiterate the title of the conference, "Management of Pharyngitis." Note that it does not state specifically group A streptococcal pharyngitis. Appropriately, discussions included consideration of other causes of sore throat, especially *Hemophilus influenzae*. Data were presented that confirm the striking drop in incidence of acute rheumatic fever. Dr. Stollerman quoted current rates of 200–400 cases per year per 100,000 in areas of Capetown and Durban, South Africa. In the United States in 1935–36, the overall rate for primary rheumatic fever was 28 per 100,000 per year (Gordis). In Baltimore, rates for first attacks among five- to 19-year-old blacks decreased from 20.2 to 10.8 per 100,000 per year between 1960–64 and 1968–70. The decline occurred primarily in those census tracts in which the "Child and Youth Program" provided ready access to comprehensive care. Most strikingly, rates in Baltimore among blacks dropped to 0.5 per 100,000 per year in 1977–81. Dr. Bisno added similar data; a rate among blacks in Nashville of 55.5 per 100,000 per year in 1963–69 and 47 per 100,000 per year in New York City (Manhattan) in 1963–65. Yet in Memphis in 1977–81, the rate among blacks in Memphis/Shelby County was 1.2 per 100,000 per year and only 3.7 among the inner-city black population. These compare with rates of 2.3 per 100,000 per year among school-age individuals in Malmo, Sweden, in 1957–61. The key question is how much of this drop in incidence relates to the host, how much to the agent, and how much to the environment, including treatment. Analysis of the data presented suggests that treatment must be considered to be an important factor in the drop in incidence of acute rheumatic fever (Table 18–1). At least treatment could account for the decrease.

I came to this conference without preconceived conclusions; however, I was prepared to accept that the risk of penicillin reactions of one to five percent, with one in 10,000 being anaphylactic, might now exceed the risk of significant long-term disability from acute rheumatic fever and that the justification for treatment of group A streptococcal pharyngitis would be the prevention of suppurative complications and a possible shortening of the clinical course. From the data presented and the discussions, I am

TABLE 18-1. Analysis of Treatment or No Treatment of Sore Throats under Circumstances of Epidemic or Endemic Acute Rheumatic Fever

|  | Adults | Children |
|---|---|---|
| Number of sore throats | 100,000 | 100,000 |
| Percentage group A strep | 9-10 | 20-25 |
| Number sore throats with group A strep cultured | 10,000 | 25,000 |
| Percentage carriers | 50 | 50 |
| Number of sore throats minus carriers | 5,000 | 12,500 |
| Treatment |  |  |
|   Percentage of failures | 10 | 10 |
|   Number of treatment failures | 500 | 1,250 |
|   Cases of ARF per 100,000 |  |  |
|     Epidemic (2.1%)* | 10.5 | 26.2 |
|     Endemic (0.18%)** | 0.9 | 2.3[1] |
| No treatment |  |  |
|   Number of sore throats at risk | 5,000 | 12,500 |
|   Cases of ARF per 100,000 |  |  |
|     Epidemic (2.1%) | 105 | 262[2] |
|     Endemic (0.18%) | 9 | 22.5[3] |

*Rate of 2.1% from Warren Air Force Base
**Rate of 0.18% from Chicago Children's Memorial Hospital
[1]Rates of 0.9-2.3 per 100,000 approximate current rates in U.S. cities
[2]Rates of 100-260 per 100,000 approximate current rates in areas of South Africa
[3]Rates of 9-22 per 100,000 are intermediate between epidemic and endemic with treatment

forced to conclude that diagnosis and treatment of strepto-coccal pharyngitis may be an important factor in the decline of acute rheumatic fever. This is not to say that revision of current recommendations is not appropriate in terms of benefits and costs.

I would conclude that the following changes in strategies in approaching the patient with sore throat seem appropri-ate:

1. There should be more selectivity or targeting in per-forming initial cultures.
   a. Strategies should be developed and tested by age group, for example, culturing only patients between five to 17.
   b. Eliminate screening of asymptomatic individuals for group A streptococci, including family contacts.

2. Eliminate follow-up cultures.

3. There is no need for more sophisticated diagnostic procedures unless they enable differentiation between streptococcal infection and carriage.

4. Studies should be initiated to evaluate alternative agents that might both eradicate group A streptococci as well as provide symptomatic relief of sore throats due to other agents.

5. Continue the recommendation to culture sore throats (being cognizant of 1.)
   a. If positive, treat with intramuscular benzathine penicillin G or oral phenoxymethyl penicillin for ten days.
   b. Emphasize the importance of discontinuation of treatment if cultures are negative, since false-negative cultures are not epidemiologically impor-tant.

# Part Two:
# Reflections on the Conference

# 19

# Microbiologic Diagnosis of Group A Streptococcal Pharyngitis

*John A. Washington, M.D.*

Throat culture remains the principal technique for diagnosis of group A streptococcal pharyngitis because of the relative nonspecificity of clinical signs and symptoms of the disease and despite the fact that isolation of group A streptococci represents colonization or a carrier state, rather than disease, in roughly half of the patients examined. Throat cultures are simple to perform and provide accurate results, provided personnel have received proper training and follow recommended procedures.

## COLLECTION AND TRANSPORT

Either Dacron- or cotton-tipped swabs are suitable for obtaining specimens when cultures can be inoculated promptly. Breese and others have shown that the survival of group A streptococci was better in dried Dacron swabs than in dried cotton swabs that had been stored for four days at room temperature [1]; however, these results must be interpreted with caution, since it has also been shown that the survival of group A streptococci is reduced by heat and humidity [1,2]. In general, the recovery of streptococci from cotton-, Dacron-, and calcium alginate-tipped swabs under usual storage and transport conditions is equivalent. Regardless, however, of the type of swab used, it is suggested that a transport medium (Stuart's or Amies') be used for the swab when the anticipated storage and transit time is between two and 24 hours and that a silica gel or dry filter paper transport system be used if the swab is expected to be in transit for more than a day. Inexpensive swab-transport medium systems are commercially available from many sources, as are the ingredients for silica gel transport systems.

The reported difference in recovery of group A streptococci from duplicate throat swabs varies considerably but was found by Kaplan et al. [3] to be only 6% among patients with clinically overt pharyngitis. Obviously, accuracy of the procedure is highly dependent upon the training and experience of the person obtaining the specimen and how thoroughly the tonsils and posterior pharynx are swabbed. The positive culture for most discordant pairs have yielded small numbers of colonies of group A streptococci, suggesting that there is a high proportion of carriers in this group of patients [3]. Nonetheless, Kaplan et al. [3] did find that about half of the clinically overt cases with discordant throat culture results later showed an antibody rise. Although duplicate cultures will increase the detection of group A streptococci by as much as 10% in both carriers and in those with clinically overt disease, practicality and cost considerations ordinarily limit cultures to single swabs.

Throat cultures are sometimes performed as a "test-of-cure" upon completion of therapy for streptococcal pharyngitis. Since failure to eradicate the organism usually occurs in 5% to 10% of cases, the laboratory staff is often asked to interpret the significance of this finding or to perform antimicrobial susceptibility tests of such isolates. According to Kaplan [4], there is neither any compelling reason for routinely reculturing all patients treated for streptococcal pharyngitis nor for administering repeated courses of antibiotics to patients who continue to harbor group A streptococci despite adequate antibiotic therapy.

CULTURE TECHNIQUES

Medium

Essential to the cultivation of group A streptococci is an enriched infusion agar medium (for example, soybean-casein digest [tryptic or trypticase soy] agar) incorporating animal red blood cells. The medium must be free of reducing sugars that can inhibit beta-hemolysis. Defibrinated sheep blood is mixed on a 5% vol/vol basis in sterile, molten (50° C) agar and poured to a depth of 4 mm in sterile 100 mm petri dishes. This amounts to 20 ml of constituted medium per 15 × 100 mm petri dish. If the layer of medium is too thin, alpha-hemolytic colonies may appear beta-hemo-lytic, and if it is too thick, beta-hemolytic colonies may appear nonhemolytic. The final concentration of blood is not critical and can vary from 3% to 10%. Commercially prepared sheep blood agar plates are widely available from many sources.

Sheep blood contains an inhibitor of *Haemophilus haemo-lyticus* that is indigenous to the upper respiratory tract and growth of which may be confused with that of beta-hemolytic streptococci. Human blood supports the growth of *H. haemolyticus* and may contain antibiotics, antibodies, and citrate (used as anticoagulant), which are inhibitory to the growth of group A streptococci.

All media should be dated when prepared or received in the laboratory and should also have an expiration date. In general, prepared media should be stored at 2° C to 8° C to reduce evaporation of water from plates and should be used within three months of preparation. Samples of each new lot of sheep blood agar plates should be tested prior to use with controls of known positive and negative reactivity. Although a stock culture of a group A streptococcus is a suitable positive control for sheep blood agar, *Listeria monocytogenes* is a more sensitive indicator of beta-hemolysis.

Generic equivalence in performance of blood agar media produced by different manufacturers should never be presumed because of proprietary variations in supplementa-tion of the basal medium. These variations, which are not indicated on the product label, may not be apparent on quality control testing of the medium with stock cultures. Several years ago, for example, one major manufacturer's sheep blood agar performed perfectly satisfactorily in quality control tests in our laboratory; however, 35% of the group A streptococcal isolates from throat cultures on this medium demonstrated no beta-hemolysis until after a full two days of incubation (in contrast to only 2% of group A streptococcal isolates on another manufacturer's medium, which had been inoculated in parallel with the same swab). An assessment of the relative percentages of group A streptococcal isolates detected after incubation for one and two days, respectively, is probably another useful quality control procedure.

Selective Media

A variety of antimicrobial supplements have been used to try to make blood agar more selective for group A strep-tococci [2]. The results of evaluations of such media have not been consistently favorable. For example, Gunn et al. [5] and Kurzynski and Meise [6] obtained a higher rate of recovery of group A streptococci from sheep blood agar supplemented with 1.25 µg of trimethoprim per ml and 23.75 µg of sulfamethoxazole per ml than from unsupplemented sheep blood agar. In contrast, in a recently completed study at the Mayo Clinic (Libertin, Wold, and Washington, unpublished data), the incorporation of trimethoprim and sulfamethoxazole in sheep blood agar not only failed to provide any significant increase in recovery of group A streptococci, but it also significantly decreased zones of beta-hemolysis and delayed detection of group A streptococci (Table 19–1). The reasons for these contrasting results are unclear and may relate to differences in thymidine content of the media. Be that as it may, because of the conflicting data, sheep blood agar containing trimethoprim and sulfamethoxazole should never be substituted for unsupplemented sheep blood agar on a routine basis without a parallel clinical performance trial to determine whether its use will be helpful or detrimental.

Incubation

Although the optimal temperature of incubation is generally acknowledged to be 35° C to 37° C, the optimal atmosphere of incubation remains controversial. Anaerobic incubation is

TABLE 19-1. Effects of Sulfamethoxazole-trimethoprim (SXT) Supplementation of Sheep Blood Agar on Recovery of Group A Streptococci

| Incubation | | No. (%) of isolates from sheep blood agar | |
|---|---|---|---|
| Atmosphere | Duration (h) | Alone | Plus SXT |
| Air | 24 | 294 (16.3) | 101 (10.6) |
| | 48 | 327 (18.1) | 312 (17.3) |
| $CO_2$ (5%-10%) | 24 | 209 (11.6) | 211 (11.7) |
| | 48 | 282 (15.6) | 321 (17.8) |
| Anaerobic | 24 | 236 (13.1) | 224 (12.4) |
| | 48 | 309 (17.1) | 309 (17.1) |

recommended by some to ensure detection of group A streptococci that produce only the oxygen-labile hemolysin,
streptolysin 0. Such strains are, however, exceedingly
rare. The results shown in Table 19–1 confirm an earlier
report by Murray et al. [7] from this laboratory that
incubation in an atmosphere with 3% to 5% $CO_2$ and anaerobically does not significantly increase the rate of recovery of group A streptococci when compared with that in
an atmosphere of room air. In no instance were group A
streptococci detected only by subsurface hemolytic reactions
in areas in which the agar was stabbed with inoculum.
These data stand in contrast to those reported by Dykstra
et al. [8] and by Lauer et al. [9], who found that group A
streptococci were recovered significantly more frequently by
anaerobic than by aerobic incubation. The reasons for
these differences are not readily apparent but may be
medium-related. Both studies favoring anaerobic incubation
were performed with the same manufacturer's (BBL Microbiology Systems) trypticase soy blood agar medium, whereas
both of the studies in this laboratory were performed with
another manufacturer's (Gibco Laboratories) trypticase soy
blood agar medium.

Anaerobic incubation *may,* therefore, increase the rate of
recovery of group A streptococci. Anaerobic incubation,
however, significantly increases the rate of recovery of
non-group A beta-hemolytic streptococci [7,9] (Table 19–1).
Hence, the greater sensitivity for group A streptococci of
anaerobic incubation may not justify the extra effort and
expense required to differentiate group A from non-group A
beta-hemolytic streptococci [9].

Regardless of what atmosphere of incubation is used, a
small percentage ($\leq 5\%$) of group A streptococci will be
detected only by extending the period of incubation from 24
to 48 hours [7,9] (Table 19–1). Also, regardless of whether this small additional yield is clinically important, the
additional day of incubation may, as was discussed previously, be an important quality control check on the medium.

IDENTIFICATION

Presumptive Identification

Group A and non-group A beta-hemolytic streptococci are
most frequently differentiated presumptively with the bacitracin disk differentiation test. When evaluated in purified
subcultures, between 0% and 5% of group A streptococci
have failed to be inhibited by the bacitracin disk and

between 3% and 17% of non-group A beta-hemolytic streptococci have been inhibited by the bacitracin disk. These
differences in false-negative and false-positive results are
largely methodologically related to variations in disk content
of bacitracin, inoculum size, and interpretation of zone
diameters of inhibition.

The bacitracin test must be performed with the differential (0.04 unit) disk, rather than with that used for
susceptibility testing. The test must be restricted to
beta-hemolytic streptococci since many alpha-hemolytic
streptococci, including pneumococci, are inhibited by bacitracin. The inoculum may be prepared by subculturing one
or two colonies from the primary culture plate into 2 ml of
broth, mixing well, dipping a cotton swab into the broth
suspension, and expressing excess fluid from the swab
against the side of the tube. After streaking the swab
across the surface of a blood agar plate and applying the
bacitracin disk to the agar surface, the plate is incubated
overnight at 35° C. Any zone of inhibition whatsoever is
considered presumptively positive for group A streptococci.
Although 10 mm has been suggested by some as the minimum zone diameter of inhibition indicative of group A
streptococci, studies in this laboratory have shown that
only 3% of bacitracin-susceptible beta-hemolytic streptococci
had zones of less than 10 mm [10]. Any size zone of
inhibition should, therefore, be considered as presumptive
evidence of isolation of group A streptococci.

Application of bacitracin disks to the primary culture
plates has been recommended by some as a means of reducing the time required to achieve presumptive identification
of group A streptococci. In a previous study from this
laboratory, bacitracin disks placed in the center of the area
of initial inoculation and in the second area streaked on the
primary culture plates detected slightly more than half of
all group A streptococcal isolates. The reasons for not
detecting the remaining group A streptococcal isolates were
the presence of too few colonies in the vicinity of the disk,
overgrowth by other bacteria around the disk, and the lack
of any detectable zone of inhibition around the disk.
Overgrowth by colonies of bacteria other than group A
streptococci can be inhibited by applying a trimethoprim
(1.25 µg)-sulfamethoxazole (23.75 µg) or SXT disk adjacent
to the bacitracin disk in the area of initial inoculation on
the blood agar plate. By using this approach, Baron and
Gates [11] were able to detect 75% of group A streptococci
after overnight incubation. The 25% increment in detection
rate in their study corresponds with that not detected in
our study because of bacterial overgrowth. Kurzynski et

al. [12] accomplished the same goal by applying bacitracin disks to blood agar plates containing trimethoprim and sulfamethoxazole.

Definitive Identification

Definitive identification of group A streptococci depends on extracting the group-specific C polysaccharide and reacting it with group A-specific antiserum. The antigen may be extracted with hot HCL, hot formamide, nitrous acid, enzymes, or by autoclaving. Techniques for determining antigen-antibody reactions include capillary and gel diffusion precipitin tests, counterimmunoelectrophoresis, coagglutination, latex agglutination, and immunofluorescence. The technique selected for use in any laboratory is primarily contingent upon technical and cost considerations.

Immunofluorescence has been used for many years to examine stained sediments of two- to five-hour broth cultures of throat swabs. In our experience, 2% to 4% of culture-positive swabs have been negative by immunofluorescence; the converse (positive immunofluorescence, negative culture) has occurred in less than 1% of instances. Detection of group A streptococci is poor by immunofluorescent antibody staining of smears made directly from throat swabs.

El Kholy et al. [13] used a modified nitrous acid extraction microtechnique and rapid capillary precipitin reaction to test throat scrapings and detected group A streptococci in 85% of culture-positive patients. The direct method failed to detect group A streptococci in throat scrapings of patients whose cultures yielded 15 or fewer colonies of the organism. Similar results have been reported for throat swabs with a micronitrous acid extraction-coagglutination technique by Slifkin and Gil [14] and by Gerber [15]. Gerber [15] reported the test as 78% sensitive and 98% specific. A single swab can be tested in approximately 20 minutes [14], while a batch of 18 swabs can be tested in approximately one hour [15]. Edwards et al. [16] reported similar levels of sensitivity and specificity with a latex agglutination test of throat gargle material.

In sum, there are a variety of acceptable extraction procedures and techniques for definitively identifying group A streptococci in cultures. Some of these techniques have been evaluated for direct testing of throat secretions and have generally lacked sensitivity when small numbers of group A streptococci have been isolated in parallel cultures. Although heavy growth of group A streptococci is more frequently associated with clinically overt cases of strepto-coccal pharyngitis and light growth with carriers, this correlation is far from perfect and is highly dependent on the vigor with which the throat is swabbed, to mention only one of several factors. Hence, one must be very cautious about dismissing cultures yielding few colonies of group A streptococci as being clinically insignificant.

Considerable effort is being devoted to developing en-zyme immunoassays for detecting group A streptococci. Preliminary results of clinical trials appear encouraging; however, further studies are needed to define the sensi-tivity, specificity, reproducibility, practicality, and cost effectiveness of this and other novel approaches.

## Identification of Other Bacteria

The role of non-group A beta-hemolytic streptococci remains unclear. Foodborne epidemics related to groups C and G streptococci have been reported [17,18], and non-group A beta-hemolytic streptococci have been more frequently isolated from nonepidemic cases with pharyngitis in various populations in Louisiana and Mississippi [19] and in college students [20,21]. Glezen et al. [21] isolated non-group A beta-hemolytic streptococci from 0.2% of asymptomatic college students and from 10.8% of students with pharyngitis. In contrast, Hable et al. [22] isolated non-group A beta-hemolytic streptococci from 6.7% of 490 children with upper respiratory infection and 6.3% of 490 matched controls. Over a three-year period, Murray et al. [23] found that group A streptococci represented between 25% and 68% of beta-hemolytic streptococci isolated from throat swabs at the Mayo Clinic. This fluctuation was entirely attributable to seasonal variations in the recovery of group A streptococci.

Whether non-group A beta-hemolytic streptococci can cause clinically overt nonepidemic upper respiratory in-fection remains uncertain. Kaplan et al. [4] isolated non-group A beta-hemolytic streptococci from 13% of chil-dren presenting with signs and/or symptoms of pharyngitis; however, fewer than 5% of this group and of another group from whom no beta-hemolytic streptococci were isolated experienced a significant rise in antibody titer (ASO and anti-DNase B), in contrast to significant rises in anti-body titer in 27% of a group that was culture-positive and cured with a single course of therapy and in 54% of another group that was culture-positive and cured only after a second course of therapy. The failure of non-group A beta-hemolytic streptococci to elicit an antibody response in this study differs from that following a foodborne epidemic of group G streptococcal pharyngitis at a college in which Hill et al. [18] demonstrated a significant antibody (ASO) rise in 53% of 38 students who were culture-positive.

In sum, there are conflicting epidemiologic data on the etiologic role of non-group A beta-hemolytic streptococci in nonepidemic pharyngitis. Interpretation of their presence cannot be made reliably unless their incidence in matched controls in a particular community is known. Concurrent infection with other recognized etiologic agents occurs frequently [21], and significant rises in antibody appear to occur rarely. Nonsuppurative sequelae of nonepidemic non-group A beta-hemolytic streptococcal upper respiratory infection have not been recognized. Moreover, there are no convincing data that antibiotic therapy is required in such cases. Consequently, identification of non-group A beta-hemolytic streptococci in throat cultures does not appear to be necessary on a routine basis and, if reported, may lead to unnecessary antibiotic treatment. On the other hand, identification of such isolates is indicated in suspected foodborne epidemics so that appropriate epidemiologic control measures can be taken. Because so few such outbreaks have been recognized, appropriate measures for clinical management of cases have not been determined. No sequelae were identified among the college students studied by Hill et al. [18]; however, Duca et al. [17] reported that a third of their cases developed acute glomerulonephritis.

Other than group A streptococci, bacteria of established etiologic importance in tonsillopharyngitis include *Bordetella pertussis, Corynebacterium diphtheriae,* and *Neisseria gonorrhoeae.* Organisms such as *Staphylococcus aureus, Streptococcus pneumoniae, Haemophilus influenzae,* the Enterobacteriaceae, and *Pseudomonas aeruginosa* often transiently colonize the upper respiratory tract but have no established etiologic role in tonsillopharyngitis and should not be routinely reported. The viridans streptococci, diphtheroids, coagulase-negative staphylococci, nonpathogenic neisseriae, and a great variety of gram-positive and gram-negative anaerobic cocci and rods constitute normal oropharyngeal flora and certainly should not be reported.

The persistence of group A streptococci in throat cultures following one or more courses of penicillin often prompts a request for the laboratory staff to determine whether any *S. aureus* which are present in the throat culture produce beta-lactamase. Although initially suggested as a cause of treatment failure [24], the presence of beta-lactamase-producing *S. aureus* has subsequently been shown not to correlate with the failure of penicillin to eradicate group A streptococci from the throat [25,26]. This issue today is further complicated by the frequent occurrence of beta-lactamase-producing coagulase-negative staphylococci, *H. influenzae, Branhamella catarrhalis,* and anaerobic gram-negative rods in the oropharynx. Hence, any request to search for beta-lactamase-producing *S. aureus* as a cause of treatment failure is overly simplistic and not supported by the available evidence.

In summary, the routine throat culture report can simply state the presence or absence of growth of group A streptococci. Unless specimen collection is performed in a consistent, reproducible manner by one or two properly trained persons, reporting growth in semiquantitative terms (for example, many, moderate, few, or 4+, 3+, 2+, 1+) is probably meaningless and potentially misleading. Reporting the presence of non-group A beta-hemolytic streptococci does not appear to be justified on a routine basis; however, one should be alert to the possibility of foodborne epidemics of pharyngitis and the need to incubate cultures in such instances under anaerobic conditions to enhance the recovery of non-group A beta-hemolytic streptococci [7–9] (Table 19–1).

## ANTIBIOTIC SUSCEPTIBILITY TESTS

Group A streptococci are uniformly susceptible to penicillin and other beta-lactam antibiotics. Penicillin tolerance (that is, MBC/MIC ratio of 8 to 32) was reported by Allen and Sprunt [27]; however, the significance of their findings is difficult to determine since their studies were performed with a stationary phase inoculum (overnight broth culture), which is more resistant to killing than that from a logarithmic phase culture [28]. Penicillin-resistant and penicillin-tolerant mutants have been isolated from mutagenized group A streptococci by Gutmann and Tomasz [29]; however, such bacteria have not yet been recognized among natural isolates.

Resistance of group A streptococci to erythromycin and tetracycline has recently been reported by Bourbeau and Campos [30] in Philadelphia as 3% and 5%, respectively, and by Haddy et al. [31] in Saginaw, Michigan, to be 4.3% and 7.8%, respectively; however, over 60% of strains tested by Maruyama et al. [32] in Asahikawa, Japan, were resistant to erythromycin, lincomycin, chloramphenicol, and tetracycline. Resistance in such instances is commonly plasmid-borne [33], in contrast with that reported by Gutmann and Tomasz [29] in laboratory mutants and which appears to be related to decreased affinity of penicillin-binding proteins for penicillin.

In conclusion, susceptibility testing of group A streptococci to penicillin and other beta-lactam antibiotics is not indicated at this time; however, when the use of penicillins is contraindicated, susceptibility testing to erythromycin, tetracycline, and clindamycin should be performed.

## A CLINICAL MICROBIOLOGIST'S CONFERENCE PERSPECTIVE

Throat culture for group A streptococci remains the standard for the diagnosis of group A streptococcal pharyngitis; however, roughly 50% of children with positive throat cultures never develop any serologic evidence of infection. Therefore, although the false-negative rate of throat cultures is low in patients with serologically proven group A streptococcal pharyngitis, the false-positive rate is substantial. Moreover, the development and use of more sensitive or selective culture methods or other detection techniques probably only increase the rate of detection of carriers, who, according to studies by Kaplan and his coworkers, do not appear at risk of developing rheumatic fever and do not require antibiotic therapy. The declining incidence of rheumatic fever in the United States to rates below 1/100,000 population further reduces the need or justification for more sensitive detection techniques. It appears, therefore, that what is really needed is a rapid, simple, and specific test for detecting group A streptococci in patients with disease only or for differentiating between those with disease and those who are carriers. Whether and how this might be accomplished remains highly speculative and uncertain. Although it appears likely that simple and inexpensive antigen detection systems with sensitivity and specificity rates equivalent to those of cultures will become available in the near future, such devices appear unlikely to resolve the fundamental problem of detecting excessively high rates of carriers.

It now appears unnecessary to perform throat cultures after a course of antibiotics as a "test-of-cure," or to subject patients whose throat cultures remain positive following treatment to repeated courses of antibiotics, unless signs and symptoms suggestive of group A streptococcal pharyngitis persist. The explanation for bacteriologic treatment failure remains unknown but is unrelated to the emergence of resistance to penicillin by group A streptococci or to the presence of beta-lactamase-producing staphylococci in the throat. Whether the presence of other beta-lactamase-producing bacteria, such as *Haemophilus, Branhamella,* or *Bacteroides,* adversely affect treatment with penicillin remains unknown. Be that as it may, cultures of asymptomatic individuals and family contacts, susceptibility testing of group A streptococci to penicillin, and the isolation and identification of beta-lactamase-producing staphylococci are *not* warranted at this time. Because, however, up to 10% of group A streptococci in this country and over 60% of those in Japan are resistant to erythromycin, tetracycline, and lincomycin, the susceptibility of strains to these antibiotics should be tested when penicillin therapy is contraindicated. Certainly, continued surveillance for emerging patterns of resistance is necessary.

A related and disturbing issue that emerged at the conference was the finding in a CDC survey that 42% of family practitioners who administered antibiotics prior to the availability of throat culture results failed to discontinue therapy if the culture proved negative. Although the proportion of pediatricians admitting to this practice was only 26%, the implications of this antibiotic abuse are obvious and should stimulate educational efforts to correct the situation. An important corollary to this effort should be undertaken by clinical laboratories to expedite processing of throat cultures and reporting of results. According to the CDC survey, fees charged for throat cultures ranged from $8.45 to $13.80. The implementation of more costly detection or identification devices certainly appears unwarranted, particularly if such devices are supplementary to cultures. The economic and clinical consequences of using a rapid antigen detection system and reserving culture for antigen-negative swabs must be studied carefully. Also, what appears to be a rapid test for the microbiology laboratory may not be when it is compared to the time occupied by an office visit. In other words, if the test cannot be completed while the patient is in the office, it is unlikely to alter current therapeutic practices.

A major unresolved issue remains the possible etiologic roles in pharyngitis of organisms other than group A streptococci, gonococci, diphtheria and pertussis bacilli, mycoplasmas, and viruses. Although clearly involved in a few well-documented foodborne epidemics of pharyngitis, the association of non-group A beta-hemolytic streptococci with nonepidemic pharyngitis is at best circumstantial. Similar arguments regarding *Haemophilus influenzae* persist, despite the lack of supporting data. Anecdotal reports of resolution of pharyngitis following treatment with penicillins of patients from whom non-group A beta-hemolytic streptococci were isolated provide unconvincing evidence of their role in causing the disease and do not exclude the possible etiologic role of other microorganisms, especially since most episodes of pharyngitis spontaneously resolve rapidly without specific antimicrobial therapy. The absence to date of specific antibody markers or sequelae of pharyngeal non-group A beta-hemolytic streptococcal "infection" complicates this issue considerably but will, it is hoped, stimulate further research into the etiology of pharyngitis in patients from whom established agents cannot be isolated. At any rate, except in suspected epidemic situations, there appear to be no compelling reasons for throat culture reports to state anything more than whether or not group A streptococci were present. Reporting of other species confers a sense of their importance and places the burden of proof on the laboratory that specific treatment of such species is clinically important.

REFERENCES

1. Breese, B. B., and C. B. Hall. 1978. Beta hemolytic streptococcal diseases. Boston: Houghton Mifflin, 9–33.
2. Facklam, R. R. 1976. A review of the microbiological techniques for the isolation and identification of streptococci. *CRC Crit Rev Clin Lab Sci* 6:287–317.
3. Kaplan, E. L., R. Couser, B. B. Huwe, C. McKay, and L. W. Wannamaker. 1979. Significance of quantitative salivary cultures for group A and non-group A β-hemolytic streptococci in patients with pharyngitis and in their family contacts. *Pediatrics* 64:904–12.
4. Kaplan, E. L., A. S. Gastanaduy, and B. B. Huwe. 1981. The role of the carrier in treatment failures after antibiotic therapy for group A streptococci in the upper respiratory tract. *J Lab Clin Med* 98:326–35.
5. Gunn, B. A., D. K. Ohashi, C. A. Gaydos, and E. S. Holt. 1977. Selective and enhanced recovery of group A and B streptococci from throat cultures with sheep blood agar containing sulfamethoxazole and trimethoprim. *J Clin Microbiol* 5:650–55.
6. Kurzynski, T. A., and C. K. Meise. 1979. Evaluation of sulfamethoxazole-trimethoprim blood agar plates for recovery of group A streptococci from throat cultures. *J Clin Microbiol* 9:189–93.
7. Murray, P. R., A. D. Wold, C. A. Schreck, and J. A. Washington II. 1976. Effects of selective media and

atmosphere of incubation on the isolation of group A streptococci. *J Clin Microbiol* 4:54–56.

8. Dykstra, M. A., J. C. McLaughlin, and R. C. Bartlett. 1979. Comparison of media and techniques for detection of group A streptococci in throat swab specimens. *J Clin Microbiol* 9:236–38.

9. Lauer, B. A., L. B. Reller, and S. Mirrett. 1983. Effect of atmosphere and duration of incubation on primary isolation of group A streptococci from throat cultures. *J Clin Microbiol* 17:338–40.

10. Murray, P. R., A. D. Wold, M. M. Hall, and J. A. Washington II. 1976. Bacitracin differentiation for presumptive identification of group A β-hemolytic streptococci: comparison of primary and purified plate testing. *J Pediatr* 89:576–79.

11. Baron, E. J., and J. W. Gates. 1979. Primary plate identification of group A beta-hemolytic streptococci utilizing a two-disk technique. *J Clin Microbiol* 10:80–84.

12. Kurzynski, T., C. Meise, R. Daggs, and A. Helstad. 1979. Improved reliability of the primary plate bacitracin test on throat cultures with sulfamethoxazole-trimethoprim blood agar plates. *J Clin Microbiol* 9:144–46.

13. El Kholy, A., R. Facklam, G. Sabri, and J. Rotta. 1978. Serological identification of group A streptococci from throat scrapings before culture. *J Clin Microbiol* 8:725–28.

14. Slifkin, M., and G. M. Gil. 1982. Serogrouping of β-hemolytic streptococci from throat swabs with nitrous acid extraction and the Phadebact Streptococcus Test. *J Clin Microbiol* 15:187–89.

15. Gerber, M. A. 1983. Micronitrous acid extraction-coaggulatination test for rapid diagnosis of streptococcal pharyngitis. *J Clin Microbiol* 17:170–71.

16. Edwards, E. A., I. A. Phillips, and W. C. Suiter. 1982. Diagnosis of group A streptococcal infections directly from throat specimens. *J Clin Microbiol* 15:481–83.

17. Duca, E., G. Teodorovici, C. Radu, A. Vita, P. Talasman-Niculescu, E. Bernescu, C. Feldi, and V. Rosca. 1969. A new nephritogenic streptococcus. *J Hyg* (Camb) 67:691–98.

18. Hill, H. R., G. G. Caldwell, E. Wilson, D. Hager, and R. A. Zimmerman. 1969. Epidemic of pharyngitis due to streptococci of Lancefield group G. *Lancet* 2:371–74.

19. Mogabgab, W. J. 1970. Beta-hemolytic streptococcal and concurrent infections in adults and children with respiratory disease, 1958 to 1969. *Ann Rev Resp Dis* 102:23–34.

20. Evans, A. S., and E. C. Dick. 1964. Acute

pharyngitis and tonsillitis in University of Wisconsin students. *JAMA* 190:699–708.

21. Glezen, W. P., G. W. Fernald, and J. A. Lohr. 1975. Acute respiratory disease of university students with special reference to the etiologic role of *Hespesvirus hominis*. *Am J Epidemiol* 101:111–21.

22. Hable, K. A., J. A. Washington II, and E. C. Herrmann, Jr. 1971. Bacterial and viral throat flora: comparison of findings in children with acute upper respiratory tract disease and in healthy controls during winter. *Clin Pediatr* 10:199–203.

23. Murray, P. R., A. D. Wold, and J. A. Washington II. 1977. Recovery of group A and nongroup A β-hemolytic streptococci from throat swab specimens. *Mayo Clin Proc* 52:81–84.

24. Kundsin, R. B., and J. M. Miller. 1964. Significance of the *Staphylococcus aureus* carrier state in the treatment of disease due to group A streptococci. *N Engl J Med* 271:1395–97.

25. Quie, P. G., H. C. Pierce, and L. W. Wannamaker. 1966. Influence of penicillinase-producing staphylococci on the eradication of group A streptococci from the upper respiratory tract by penicillin treatment. *Pediatrics* 37:467–76.

26. Markowitz, M., I. Kramer, E. Goldstein, A. Perlman, D. Klein, R. Kramer, and M. L. Blue. 1967. Persistence of group A streptococci as related to penicillinase-producing staphylococci: comparison of penicillin V potassium and sodium nafcillin. *J Pediatr* 71:132–37.

27. Allen, J. L., and K. Sprunt. 1978. Discrepancy between minimum inhibitory and minimum bactericidal concentrations of penicillin for group A and group B β-hemolytic streptococci. *J Pediatr* 93:69–71.

28. Kim, K. S., and B. F. Anthony. 1981. Importance of bacterial growth phase in determining minimal bactericidal concentrations of penicillin and methicillin. *Antimicrob Agents Chemother* 19:1075–77.

29. Gutmann, L., and A. Tomasz. 1982. Penicillin-resistant and penicillin-tolerant mutants of group A streptococci. *Antimicrob Agents Chemother* 22:128–36.

30. Bourbeau, P., and J. M. Campos. 1982. Current antibiotic susceptibility of group A β-hemolytic streptococci. *J Infect Dis* 145:916.

31. Haddy, R. I., R. C. Gordon, L. Shamiyeh, R. Wofford, L. Fechner, and E. Sahanek. 1982. Erythromycin resistance in group A beta-hemolytic streptococci. *Pediatr Infect Dis* 1:236–38.

32. Maruyama, S., H. Yoshioka, K. Fujita, M. Taki-

moto, and Y. Satake. 1979. Sensitivity of group A strep-tococci to antibiotics. *Am J Dis Child* 133:1143–45.

33. Clewell, D. B. 1981. Plasmids, drug resistance, and gene transfer in the gene *Streptococcus*. *Microbiol Rev* 45:409–36.

# 20

# The Disappearance of Rheumatic Fever: Why?

*Edward A. Mortimer, M.D.,*
*and Harold B. Houser, M.D.*

Beginning in the early 1950s, major efforts have been made to control rheumatic fever in the United States, largely under the leadership of the American Heart Association and the military. The demonstrated efficacy of antimicrobial drugs, especially penicillin, in primary and secondary prevention, offered promise of success in these efforts. At present, after three decades, it is clear that rates of rheumatic fever have declined remarkably, and the disease is a rarity in this country. Anecdotal impressions that this is so are confirmed by population-based data from Baltimore and Nashville and from the military services, as well as by mortality figures [1].

It is tempting to ascribe this salutary situation to the development of penicillin and its widespread use in regimens proved to be efficacious in preventing rheumatic fever. But there is evidence that at least some of the decline in morbidity and mortality from rheumatic fever may be due to ill-defined factors other than antimicrobial drugs. Prior to the development of penicillin and its use, there was evidence that the disease was declining in severity, as measured by the extent of cardiac sequelae [2]. The possibility that part or all of this decline was apparent rather than real, due to the recognition and inclusion of milder cases as diagnostic criteria improved, must be considered. But in Sweden, mortality data have indicated that mortality ascribed to rheumatic heart disease was declining as rapidly prior to the advent of penicillin as afterwards [3]. Accordingly, there is question about the unique role of penicillin in controlling rheumatic fever.

The importance of the answer to this question lies in its impact on any consideration of modifications of the current recommendations for prevention of rheumatic fever. If penicillin is indeed largely responsible for the decline in rheumatic fever, relaxation of recommendations may result in recrudescence of unacceptable rates of rheumatic fever. If it is not, easing of recommendations may reduce health care costs and inconvenience without increases in rheumatic fever and rheumatic heart disease.

In this symposium, Gordis has offered three possible explanations for the decline in rheumatic fever: altered host factors; changes in the organism; and environmental factors. Gordis discards alterations in host factors on the basis that such would only be expected to take place over generations, and believes that the demonstrable effect of well-designed programs for control of streptococcal infections and rheumatic fever is evidence of a major role for penicillin. The contributions of changes in such environmental factors as nutrition, socioeconomic conditions, and the like cannot be ascertained.

But recognition and treatment of the responsible group A streptococcal respiratory infections cannot be the entire explanation, for the reason that up to 40% of group A streptococcal infections that cause rheumatic fever are inapparent or sufficiently mild to cause no concern [4]. Further, it is unlikely that optimum management even of *clinical* streptococcal pharyngitis is carried out by all physicians [5]. Thus, it seems likely that the remarkable decline in rheumatic fever exceeds that which would be expected just from recognition and treatment of clinical streptococcal disease in individual patients and families. Why might this have occurred?

In trying to answer this question, advantage may be taken of known interactions between the functional anatomy of the group A streptococcus and its epidemiological characteristics. It is our hypothesis that the virulence and transmissability of group A streptococci in the United States have been altered by the environment in at least one and possibly two ways.

Virulence, including transmissability, of the group A streptococcus is to a large extent dependent upon the M protein content of its cell wall. In man it has been shown that strains of group A streptococci rich in M protein infect others more readily than variants producing less of this antigen. In mice inoculated intraperitoneally, lethality is usually dependent on M protein production of the organism.

*In vitro* studies of phagocytosis of the group A streptococcus show that the M protein content of the organism relates directly to its survival.

What factors influence variation in M protein production and, hence, virulence? In a commonly used animal model, repeated intraperitoneal transfer of group A streptococci in mice often results in enhanced virulence as measured by logarithmic decreases in the number of organisms required for infection. This enhanced virulence is associated with increased M protein production by the organism, and probably takes place by selection for variants richer in M protein with successive mouse passage. Indeed, by repeated mouse passage, untypeable strains may revert to being typeable by the Lancefield technique.

A series of events analogous to mouse passage may occur in man. It appears that localized epidemics of group A streptococcal disease in civilian and military communities are associated with organisms of high virulence as measured by M protein production; in such single-strain outbreaks, the organisms recovered from patients are readily typeable by the Lancefield method and therefore are rich in M protein. It is logical to assume that this enhanced virulence and M protein production resulted from accelerated person-to-person transmission, with selection of more virulent strains, as occurs with the mouse model. In contrast, organisms recovered from sporadic, nonepidemic streptococcal infections are less apt to be typeable. Further, it is well known that prolonged carriage of group A streptococci in man is associated with decreased transmissability, and declining M protein production by the organism to the extent that it may no longer be typeable.

It is our hypothesis that the widespread use of penicillin may have altered the natural history and epidemiology of group A streptococcal disease by interfering with person-to-person transmission. Interference with transmission would be expected to minimize enhancement of M protein production and, hence, virulence of strains of group A streptococci that appear in a community. If this is so, the risk of acquiring a group A streptococcal infection is less at present than in the past not only because opportunities for exposure are diminished by treatment of clinical cases with an antimicrobial agent, but also because organisms of lower virulence are less apt to transmit to exposed, susceptible individuals.

If this hypothesis is valid, one would expect that strains of group A streptococci recovered from pharyngitis in recent years might be less likely to be M protein typeable than in the past. Although anecdotal impressions suggest that this may be so, the question has not been addressed directly in published reports. Strains of group A streptococci causing military outbreaks during World War II were much more likely to be M typeable than strains recovered from civilian populations subsequently, but these population groups are not comparable [6].

Examination of data from two published studies, which were conducted for other purposes but included M-typing of group A streptococci over time, does not provide evidence to support this hypothesis. In one, Quinn monitored streptococcal carriage by Nashville school children from 1953 to 1974 [7]. Nearly 54,000 cultures were obtained, of which approximately 7,000 yielded group A streptococci. The greatest population (60%) of typeable strains occurred in the first year of the study, but no subsequent trend is evident.

In Britain, Hope-Simpson [8] performed 7,448 throat cultures on patients with respiratory diseases for the years 1962–75. Of these, 353 (4.7%) yielded group A streptococci, 78% of which were from patients whose primary complaint was sore throat. M-typing was performed on 301 strains. No trend over time toward untypeability can be ascertained from the data, but the numbers are small, particularly in the later years of observation.

However, our hypothesis is supported by as yet unpublished data from Syracuse kindly provided by Feldman [9]. For the 18 years, 1950 through 1967, M-typing was performed on strains of group A streptococci recovered from specimens submitted to the health department laboratory; the vast majority of these strains was obtained from individuals with pharyngitis, and the average number of strains typed exceeded 500 annually. Typing sera employed varied little over the years, and included the vast majority of types. Proportions of group A streptococcal strains that were untypeable ranged from 10% to 37% during each of the first five years, 1950–54. Subsequently, for each of the 13 years, 1955–67, the majority of streptococcal isolates were untypeable, ranging between 50% and 77%. Pending further analysis, these results support the hypothesis.

One other longitudinal study has been conducted that has included M-typing of streptococci recovered from children with pharyngitis. Breese and colleagues have typed strains recovered from children with pharyngitis in office practice in Rochester, New York, but the typing results have not been examined with this question in mind [10]. Inasmuch as this study began in the early 1950s and continued into the 1970s, and because the strains of streptococci were recovered from individuals with clinical illnesses, it should be useful to examine these data from the stand-point of secular changes in typeability.

Until this question of whether changes in the virulence of prevalent group A streptococci have resulted from the widespread use of penicillin and other questions have been answered, we believe that caution should be observed in considering relaxation of current recommendations for the prevention of rheumatic fever by control of streptococcal infections. Recrudescence of rheumatic fever and rheumatic heart disease would be unfortunate indeed.

REFERENCES

1. Stamler, J. 1962. Cardiovascular diseases in the United States. *Amer J Cardiol* 10:319.

2. Bland, E. F. 1960. Declining severity of rheumatic fever. A comparative study of the past four decades. *N Engl J Med* 262:597.

3. Hemminki, E., and A. Paakkulainen. 1976. The effect of antibiotics on mortality from infectious diseases in Sweden and Finland. *Am J Pub Health* 66:1180.

4. Mortimer, E. A., Jr., and B. Boxerbaum. 1965. Diagnosis and treatment: Group A streptococcal infections. *Pediatrics* 36:930.

5. Grossman, B. J., and J. Stamler. 1963. Potential preventability of first attacks of acute rheumatic fever in children. *JAMA* 183:985.

6. Stollerman, G. H., A. C. Siegel, and E. E. Johnson. 1965. Variable epidemiology of streptococcal disease and the changing pattern of rheumatic fever. *Mod Concepts Cardiovasc Dis* 34:45.

7. Quinn, R. W. 1980. Hemolytic streptococci in Nashville school children. *South Med J* 73:288.

8. Hope-Simpson, R. E. 1981. *Streptococcus pyogenes* in the throat: a study in a small population, 1962–1975. *J Hyg* 87:109.

9. Feldman, H. A. 1983. Personal communication.

10. Breese, B. B. 1978. Beta-hemolytic streptococcus: Its bacteriologic culture and character. *Am J Dis Child* 132:502.

# 21

# The Chagrin Factor vs Iatromathematics: Impressions, Notes, and Reflections of an Ex-Streptococcologist

*Angelo Taranta, M.D.*

Only in America would 50 experts convene to discuss the approach to an old and disappearing disease (and persuade a pharmaceutical house to foot the bill). In the rest of the world, it would be difficult enough to do this even for a new disease or a disease of increasing incidence. It was a strange meeting, an interesting meeting, an eerie meeting, a reunion of the graduates of Rheumatic Fever University, and a wake for a disease that is not with us anymore, or just about. The disease, like a prodigal child, has gone away; not in the sense that it died, as news of its being sighted in Bombay or Cairo reach us intermittently, but, literally, "gone away," and the experts wonder why, and muse on whatever went right.

Just a few years ago I had drawn a diagram for an article tracing the history and speculating on the future of rheumatic fever. It was clear enough that rheumatic fever was decreasing, but I wondered whether the disease would linger on at the low levels then prevailing or continue to vanish, a wonderment expressed by the question marks and the dotted lines (Figure 21–1). It is now apparent that rheumatic fever *is* continuing to vanish; why is the question.

## FROM STREPTOCOCCAL NEGLECT TO STREPTOCOCCAL NEUROSIS

Dr. Milton Markowitz opened the meeting with an overview of the problem seen from his perspective of practicing

Figure 21–1. The rise and fall of rheumatic fever over time.

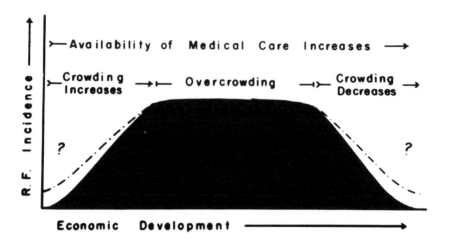

Source: From El Sadr, W., and A. Taranta. 1979. The spectrum and the specter of rheumatic fever in the 1980s. In *Clinical Immunology Update,* 183–209. E. C. Franklin, ed. New York: Elsevier.

pediatrician turned academician. Until 1950, little diagnostic attention had been focused on sore throats: The only bugaboo was diphtheria, and in fact the only time a throat culture was taken in practice was when diphtheria was suspected. Streptococci were neglected. But things started to change in the early 1950s; Markowitz, who had then just started in pediatric practice in Baltimore, happened to be consulted by the mother of a child with a sore throat; when Markowitz, without further ado, prescribed penicillin, she was plainly crestfallen; when Markowitz inquired, he learned that she had recently moved from Rochester, New York, where Dr. Breese had been her pediatrician; Breese had introduced her to the benefits of the throat culture; and now she just expected it as the hallmark of a thoughtful, up-to-date, "scientific" pediatric practice. Markowitz became a convert, and set out to proselitize, especially since information was coming in from Warren Air Force Base that penicillin treatment leading to eradication of streptococci from the throat prevented rheumatic fever. That (1950–60) was the decade of discoveries and innovations. The following decade (1960–70) was one of implementation and indoctrination, as more and more pediatricians started to culture throats, and more state health departments provided the service, often free of charge. But during the 1970s (the decade of critique and revision), the incidence of the major sequelae of streptococcal infections reached new lows, and there was a growing realization that the throat culture is not much help in distinguishing infections from carriers. A new critical attitude arose: Is the throat culture necessary? indicated? and, above all, in these money-conscious times, cost-effective? Meanwhile the general public, always a bit behind, worried about strep, often to the point of neurosis. This is especially clear now in the case of follow-up cultures, bacteriologic treatment failures, and carriers. There are patients, and there are doctors, who compulsively seek evidence of residual streptococci after treatment, even in the absence of symptoms or signs of residual or recurrent infection, and even though the usefulness of retreatment (in terms of avoiding sequelae) has never been demonstrated. Some patients, almost certainly carriers, are retreated over and over again: The anxieties of the patient and the anxieties of the doctor feed on each other to no one's benefit but the druggist's.

## THE VANISHING OF RHEUMATIC FEVER

Leon Gordis and Alan Bisno provided the evidence, recently gathered and still unpublished, of this vanishing act. In Baltimore, Gordis and his associates have collected data on rheumatic fever incidence with admittedly imperfect, but at least consistent, methods every ten years or so, over the last twenty years. From 1960–64 to 1968–70, the incidence remained constant among whites (8.6/100,000 in 1960–64, and 9.5 in 1968–70) but was halved among blacks (20.2 in 1960–64 and 10.8 in 1968–70), probably as the result of comprehensive health care programs. (However, a marked decrease occurred also in the 1920s and 1930s, when neither penicillin nor comprehensive care was around.) Over the next ten years (1970–80) the decrease gathered momentum, and involved both whites and blacks to about the same (ten-fold!) extent, reaching the 0.5/100,000/year incidence level for both groups in 1977–81. Recurrences of rheumatic fever, once a major public health problem, were reduced to only one in the city of Baltimore over a five-year period!

Bisno confirmed this striking reduction with his recent data from Memphis, where only 41 cases occurred over the five-year period 1977–81, an incidence of 0.64/100,000/year in the general population, and of 1.88/100,000/year in school-age children. Similarly low rates had been reported from Scandinavia 20 years ago (for example, 2.3/100,000 children/year in Malmö in 1957–61) and were widely attributed at the time to the homogenously high living standards prevailing in Scandinavia. And from an affluent area, Fairfax County, Virginia, Richard Schwartz reported a similar decline; while six or seven cases per year were seen in the early 1970s, years went by without a single case in the late 1970s, for a calculated rate of 0.5/100,000 per year in the 5–19-year-old age group. Rates as low as 0.2/100,000 per year in Rhode Island were mentioned and contrasted with rates as high as 65/100,000 school children/year reported as recently as 1965 in New York City. So, the impression was widespread that a roughly tenfold reduction in rheumatic fever has occurred in the United States over as short a period as ten years (1970–80). In view of this reduction, it would not be unreasonable to consider less diagnostic compulsiveness, and even a reduction of the length of treatment for streptococcal pharyngitis to 3–5 days from the current "official" ten days.

How has this change come about? The incidence of streptococcal pharyngitis hasn't really decreased, and even the percentage of typeability of isolates has remained about the same, even though mucoid strains seem to be rarer now. The conclusion seems inescapable that rheumatogenic infections have decreased whether because of a decrease of rheumatogenic types (like type 5) or because of other characteristics of the organism unrelated to serologic type.

How are things in other parts of the world? Only the roughest approximations are believable, such as the ones derived from the observation that in Israel, special wards for rheumatic fever patients were needed as recently as 15 years ago, but no longer. In India and in Africa, it is difficult to get a clear picture, in part because health services are so over-burdened that there is always a vast reservoir of unmet needs (the unmet needs are often unseen and therefore may decrease without anyone noticing), but in Cairo there is the impression of a decline, while in South Africa there isn't. A recent approximation cited by Gene Stollerman is 350 cases of rheumatic fever/100,000 children/year in the black township of Soweto. In poor sections of Santiago, Chile, there is still much rheumatic fever, and it seems to be due to a high incidence of type 5 infections. So, in the *same* day and age, there is a reported and believable greater than thousand-fold difference in attack rates of rheumatic fever in children—from a maximum, in Soweto, South Africa, of 350/100,000/year, to a minimum of 0.2/100,000/year in Rhode Island.

## THE DIAGNOSIS OF STREPTOCOCCAL PHARYNGITIS AND CHANGES THEREIN

In the face of this marked reduction of the risk of rheumatic fever, the time-honored methods of prevention have, predictably, come under fire. Renewed scrutiny has led to reexamination of the throat culture, as reviewed by Michael Gerber. Dissatisfaction with the throat culture, as outlined by Elia Ayoub, has led to a renewed interest in clinical diagnosis, as reviewed by Lewis Wannamaker, and to new experimental approaches to laboratory diagnosis, as summarized by Richard Facklam. Perhaps most importantly, this critical attitude has led to an examination of what U.S. physicians are actually doing in their practices, as reported and investigated (by the questionnaire method) by Dr. Stephen L. Cochi.

According to a survey of the National Ambulatory Care Association, sore throats are the third leading cause for visits to doctors' offices in this country. There is a lot of throat culturing, determined largely, it seems, by accidental historical factors. In Rhode Island, on the average one out of six inhabitants has a throat culture taken over a one-year period! Pediatricians, nationwide, take an average of 16 throat cultures per week; internists, three. Confronted with a patient with pharyngitis, 54% of pediatricians will take a throat culture, but only 16% of internists and 18% of general practitioners and family physicians. Sixty-five percent of pediatricians get the result of their throat culture within one day; 53% rely on the bacitracin disk method for the determination of group A versus non-group A beta-hemolytic streptococci. (But, as another participant remarked, since these data were obtained by the questionnaire method, they reflect what the physicians think they are doing, at best, or what they wish to be known as doing, at worst. What they actually do may be another story.)

As for treatment: 42% of physicians start penicillin before knowing the culture results. Seventy-four percent prefer oral penicillin; only 10% use intramuscular penicillin, and only 58% stop oral penicillin if the culture turns out to be negative. (How come? If they went to the trouble of taking the throat culture, why dismiss their results? Physicians' minds are labyrinthine.) Charges average $12 per culture with the bacitracin method.

How well can one do *without* throat cultures? Not very well, but exactly how well depends on the circumstances. In the presence of a food-borne epidemic, for instance, one can do very well, once the epidemic itself is diagnosed. In endemic circumstances, much less well. Burtis Breese proposed a nine-point scoring system, including age of the patient, season of the year, fever, sore throat, headache, abnormal pharynx, abnormal cervical glands, absence of cough, and elevation of white blood count. When used by Dr. Breese and his close associates, prediction was good when the score was definitely high or definitely low, but much less good when it was intermediate. Yet, others have had difficulty in obtaining as good as Breese's with his own scoring method; reasons for Breese's higher percentage of accurate diagnoses may have to do with the availability of culture results on other patients (that is, with knowledge of the "local epidemiology," with being aware of "what's going around"); with Breese's perceptiveness and exper- ience as a consummate pediatrician with a special interest in strep infections; with the fact that he included all upper respiratory infections in his denominator (including, that is, even infections that were obviously nonstreptococcal); and with the fact that his studies were carried out in his own private practice, which presumably afforded him the opportunity to communicate better with his patients and patients' parents than doctors do in a crowded clinic or emergency room. Finally, the inclusion of the WBC count in the data base may have helped (especially in tilting away from a diagnosis of streptococcal pharyngitis when the WBC count was low) and yet may be considered, strictly speak- ing, a laboratory rather than a clinical bit of information.

Discussion developed over the role of the streptococcus in infancy. Wannamaker recalled the classic description of "streptococcal fever, childhood type" by Powers and Boisvert, in 1944, which included a subacute constitutional reaction, mild rhinopharyngitis, thin excoriating nasal discharge, moderate- to low-grade fever of long duration (four-eight weeks), moderate cervical adenitis (sometimes suppurative), catarrhal or suppurative otitis media, oc- casional bacteremia, not infrequent suppurative compli- cations, and rare nonsuppurative sequelae. Everybody agreed that streptococcal infections occur not infrequently in the first three years of life, but that the picture of streptococcal fever just outlined is rare. Citing an ongoing study, Floyd Denny remarked that the association between clinical illness and strep acquisition is very weak during the first three years of life. In fact, taking advantage of the presence of some old-timers around the table, it was agreed that "streptococcal fever, childhood type" was rare even in Powers' and Boisvert's day. Because of the rarity of sequelae of streptococcal pharyngitis in this age group (rheumatic fever is unheard of and poststreptococcal glomerulonephritis in infants, though not rare, seems to be related more often to impetigo rather than to pharyngitis), one can certainly relax a bit. Wannamaker, however, introduced a word of caution: Maybe these early infections—which seem to be common in the developing world and may have been common here in an earlier time—precondition the host to react to a later streptococcal infection by development of rheumatic fever after three years of age.

How good are throat cultures? As many as 20% of positive cultures may be negative on a duplicate swab; but this happens mostly with weakly positive cultures. Sensitivity may be increased by anaerobic incubation; but the percentage of non-group A streps is also increased, a clear disadvantage. Should one pay attention to the number of colonies growing on a plate (and treat only those infections from which many colonies are recovered)? Perhaps yes, since there is good correlation of the number of colonies with symptoms—but perhaps no, since correlation with subsequent antibody response is questionable at best. The bacitracin disk method for distinguishing group A and non-group A streptococci continues to have a high sensitivity (95%–100%) and specificity (83%–97%). The main drawback of the throat culture remains its inability to distinguish bonafide infections from carriers.

What other laboratory means do we have to help in the diagnosis of strep infection? Nothing much, unfortunately. Direct gram-stain of a smear from a throat swab without culture or incubation found no supporters at the table: Specificity is just too low. The C-reactive protein has limited value in distinguishing streptococcal infection from streptococcal carriage (it was positive in 78% of the former and only in 53% of the latter in a study by Ed Kaplan) but practically no value in differentiating streptococcal from nonstreptococcal pharyngitis. A nitrous acid extraction method adapted as a microtechnique for analysis of throat scrapings by El Kholy in 1978 was considered tricky and essentially unsatisfactory. Coagglutination methods with antibody-coated staphylococci, ELISA, and ELISA-inhibition tests are still experimental. The latter, in addition, may detect dead as well as living group A streptococci, and thereby tilt the balance in favor of the recognition of carriers—exactly what is not wanted. The most rapid practical method of bacteriologic confirmation of clinical findings remains the immunofluorescence method applied to a broth culture, but it still involves a six-hour wait, expensive equipment, and some false-positive results (due to Fc receptors on non-group A streptococcal cells or to residual cross-reactions in incompletely absorbed antisera).

Over coffee, several participants unofficially speculated over the reasons for the persistent allure of the throat culture for a significant fraction of American physicians: "They have been brought up with it"; "It makes them feel scientific"; "Their high-class, medically sophisticated patients expect it"; "They make money with it." Only one participant gave what would have been the standard answer just a few years ago: "It's the only way to manage rationally a sore throat." Times have indeed changed. And later on, over lunch, participants searched for historical parallels—other diseases that mysteriously vanished. As Kass emphasized a decade ago, many diseases have vanished without clear relation to specific measures. Gordis remarked that the disappearance of diseases without clear relation to a cure merely reminds us that there is more to health than medicine. One is hard put now to claim a beneficial effect of improved "socioeconomic conditions," as experts once did.

Could it be that the appropriate metaphor for the interaction of rheumatogenic infection and human host is one of instability, like that of two nearly equal weights on a seesaw, whereby a small decrease of weight on one side causes a precipitous drop of the other side? Unstable equilibria are subject to catastrophes, and a catastrophe is what seems to have befallen the world of rheumatogenic infections. It may be that below a certain level of communicability, when the chain of unimpeded spread becomes shorter than a critical length, disease-producing ability collapses at a rate out of proportion to the seemingly trivial weight removed from the infection side.

## TREATMENT OF STREPTOCOCCAL PHARYNGITIS

Having exposed the uncertainties of diagnosis, the group broached the quandaries of treatment. Hugh Dillon gave an historical review, starting with Jersild's paper in 1948 on the results of treatment of scarlet fever with 150,000 units of penicillin injected intramuscularly daily for six days. The illness was shortened, and there were no complications. Further refinements were the prolongation of treatment to ten days of bactericidal activity (whether achieved by a number of injections, a number of oral doses, or a single dose of repository penicillin), and the identification of the persistence of streptococci in the throat as the most important risk factor for the development of rheumatic fever by Rammelkamp and coworkers. Six hundred thousand units of benzathine penicillin IM in small children and 1,200,000 in older children and adults became to be considered the "gold standard." An uncomfortable gold standard, to be sure. Whether this exalted state is due to the assured compliance once the needle is in, or to some other more arcane quality, we don't know, but benzathine penicillin by injection has maintained its lead compared to other methods of treatment in terms of percent bacteriology cures. Breese influenced the shift toward oral penicillin, and Markowitz noted the increased compliance with twice-a-day medication, as opposed to three or four times a day (although, as Jay Sanford remarked, it all depends on how one defines compliance: If by percentage of prescribed doses actually taken, reduction to twice-a-day may help, but is this the relevant measure or is it rather the percent of time that a bactericidal concentration of drug is maintained? Probably the latter.)

The impression exists that bacteriologic cure rates have decreased in recent years, even with benzathine penicillin injections. Why is this so? Wannamaker attributes this change to an increased proportion of carriers, who are notoriously difficult to "cure." Facklam, instead, doubts that this change is genuine, since microbiologic methods have become more sensitive over the last thirty years, and thus may detect streptococci and therefore register a "bacteriologic failure" in the same kind of throat where thirty years ago no streptococci would have been detected and therefore success would have been registered. Dillon also thinks that the bacteriologic failure rate may not have actually increased, since failure rates in the 15%–20% range may be found in the older literature also. Are other antibiotics appropriate for the treatment of streptococcal pharyngitis? Oral cephalosporins are as good as penicillin, or, according to Stollerman, even better, but of course are more expensive, and most of the experts around the table wouldn't recommend them.

Is the ten-day course still preferable to a shorter course? Schwartz cited his own 1981 comparison of ten-day vs seven-day therapy as far as eradication of streptococci from the throat is concerned. But is this still the relevant standard or, indeed, was it ever, asked Stollerman? The concept that eradication is of paramount importance, after all, was established by a single set of epidemiologic observations (by Rammelkamp's group, at Warren Air Force Base), and, Stollerman suggested, one may need to reexamine that concept. Not so, countered Wannamaker: The disease may have changed, but the Warren Air Force Base observations were sound. But, in the final analysis, what does it matter? Even if there is indeed a correlation between bacteriologic failure and rheumatic fever, since the rheumatic fever risk is now vanishingly small in most U.S. populations, the correlation is only of theoretical importance.

Ted Eickhoff reviewed the untoward effects of treatment, of which pain at the site of injection of benzathine penicillin is certainly the most common: Up to 10% of patients complain of it. It can be reduced by admixture with procaine or even with prednisolone. The most serious side effect, of course, is anaphylaxis. Its risk may be estimated at 1/100,000 injections in adults, and probably less in children (most such reports come from venereal disease clinics).

What role, if any, do organisms other than strep concomitantly present in the throat have on the outcome of treatment? There have been many contradictory findings, starting with Frank and Miller's first case report of the association of penicillinase-producing staphylococci with failure of bacteriologic cure. Anaerobes also can inactivate penicillin in the throat, and activity against anaerobes as well as streptococci is a theoretical argument in favor of using clindamycin in the treatment of streptococcal pharyngitis (treatment with clindamycin, however, is associated with up to 25% incidence of diarrhea).

## WHAT ARE CARRIERS AND SHOULD WE WORRY ABOUT THEM?

Ed Kaplan tackled this difficult topic, in which confusion reigns supreme, from the nomenclature to recommendations for management. A carrier is one with group A streptococci in his throat but without an antibody response to this organism (and therefore, the better the lab and the more antibodies examined, the more infections and the fewer carriers diagnosed). But a carrier may have had an antibody response previously, at the time of acquisition of the streptococci—he was infected first, and then became a carrier, a *convalescent* or *postinfection carrier*. This may be the most common type of carrier, and no one doubts its existence. *Chronic healthy carriers* are those who acquire a strep (or are colonized by it) on a long-term basis, but do not mount an antibody response. Finally, *contact carriers* are those who acquire streptococci without an antibody response and lose it shortly thereafter (also called *transitory* or *transient carriers*). Chronic healthy carriers are not very common, or at least have not been frequently documented, but have been reliably reported by Ayoub, Wannamaker, and others. The term "nasal carrier," however, is a misnomer since such subjects almost always are acutely infected, mount an antibody response, and therefore are not "carriers" by the general definition. In fact, nasal "carriers" were reported by Hamburger and others as being particularly contagious to contacts and therefore were considered "dangerous carriers."

Carriers, as Kaplan and Wannamaker observed, are responsible for a high proportion of treatment failures. They arrive at this conclusion because patients whose treatment fails to eradicate streptococci despite repeated courses have higher antibody titers on their initial visit, suggesting that they "had already had their infection."

## THE CHAGRIN FACTOR AND IATROMATHEMATICS

What one should do about all this, if anything, and what help we can expect from models, algorithms, computerniks, and sundry mathematics, was the subject of the last session. Alvan R. Feinstein gave easily the most stimulating and amusing talk of the meeting—a sort of introductory course on algorithms tempered by a healthy dose of skepticism. The attraction of the algorithm is that it makes us spell out our arguments; its main drawback is that not all our arguments can be spelled out. As a fringe benefit, algorithms make us realize that we don't have data on which to base our decisions; at best, they may stimulate us to collect data; at worst, they may make our decisions inappropriately rigid. Feinstein emphasized the pitfalls of transferring tests from a population of sick people to a field situation with mostly well subjects, then illustrated the difficulties of decision analysis with an amusing example drawn from culinary rather than medical experience. He convincingly demonstrated that even such a simple decision as what to do with an egg suspected of being rotten when preparing a six-egg omelet and five eggs have already been broken is almost unbearably complex. Moreover, he demonstrated that the decision that proved mathematically correct coincided with the one that intuitively "felt right": to break the suspect egg in a separate saucer, and to add it to the rest only if it proved to be fresh.

More seriously, Feinstein suggested that at the basis of many important medical decisions stood the *chagrin factor* (chagrin: disquietude or distress of mind caused by humiliation, disappointment, or failure). Physicians can tolerate much suffering—in their patients, that is, and as long as physicians don't think they have caused the suffering themselves. For instance, a physician will bear well the pain of seeing a patient develop acute rheumatic fever—but will be chagrined if that patient had come to him for management of the preceding strep infection, and he had chosen not to treat it. Likewise, the physician will tolerate a patient's anaphylactic shock from a penicillin injection given to treat streptococcal infection, but not anaphylactic shock caused by an identical injection given for nonstreptococcal pharyngitis in which the injection was not indicated—hence chagrin. Avoidance of chagrin, said Feinstein, is a strong motive in medical decisions and is often ignored by iatromathematicians.

To these arguments, Richard Tompkins answered with assurance that an algorithm is a guide, not a rule, and a flexible guide at that. To design an algorithm forces one to think problems through and to collect data, to boot. Much of medical practice, the majority perhaps, can be covered by six or seven well-designed algorithms, he said. To design an algorithm, one must collect an all-encompassing standard data base, including diagnostic studies; one must prospectively study populations for diagnostic outcomes, diagnostic yields, and corresponding costs; then one should simplify the data base, and define new algorithms to improve management and cost-effectiveness; and finally one should test the algorithms prospectively.

In the course of these operations, one should pay attention to the Kappa value, by which iatromathematicians mean the coefficient of agreement among observers for a given sign. (K is +1 in case of complete agreement and -1 in case of complete disagreement, with most cases, of course, falling in between). A decision tree will be built, but it will often be too large for practical use, and therefore will have to be pruned by eliminating the smallest or least consequential twigs. Besides pruning, the decision tree may undergo folding back, an operation whereby the cost of major branches in the tree will be calculated by adding up the costs of their respective minor branches or twigs. The advantage of designing algorithms are many, according to their designers: They make your thinking explicit; they give you a chance to separate the wheat from the chaff; their message is straightforward; they can be used in a variety of settings; and they provide well-defined standards that can be communicated to patients.

Robert H. Pantell reviewed strategies for the management of pharyngitis (which, as he underscored, are much influenced by who decides and who pays). According to a recent survey, 11% of school-age children see a doctor because of pharyngitis during a given year: a staggering patient load. The risk of no treatment is represented mainly, though not exclusively, by the attack rate of rheumatic fever, which may be calculated as 1.1-2.5/10,000 streptococcal infections. As for the risk of treatment, the Food and Drug Administration has records of only about half a dozen deaths per year in the United States from anaphylactic shock caused by penicillin, and these are mostly in adults, most of whom may have received penicillin for reasons other than pharyngitis (of course, such deaths, like anything else, may be underreported). There is a series in the literature of 314,000 benzathine penicillin injections without a single death, but this was in the military, and one may presume the existence of better precautions and greater readiness to treat anaphylactic reactions there than in the average physician's office. In venereal disease clinics, there may be one death for 94,000 patients receiving a penicillin injection. (In children, it is less than this; and following oral rather than injectable penicillin, still less.)

The goals of treatment vary according to who views them: The doctor wants to minimize his own liability (whether it be in the form of a malpractice suit or of loss of self-esteem); he may also want to maximize his income. The patient may want to minimize his own expense, but most of all he may want to avoid risks, even if the risks are small (think of the risk-averse behavior of clients of insurance companies!). Society instead may want to decrease overall health expenses.

In conclusion, Pantell remarked that there are many different costs, and many different benefits, both tangible and intangible, including increased understanding. These costs and benefits play different roles in different situations, and they may also be appraised differently. It may be that the only sure thing is that there is no single best way to deal with these problems.

The meeting was concluded by an overview and attempted synthesis by Jay Sanford. He reminded the group that measures to control communicable diseases change in response to decreases in their incidence. Changes are affected, in addition, by the efficacy as well as by the side effects of the preventive measures. For typhoid fever, for instance, the risk of disease has decreased drastically—thanks to sanitary engineering, sewage disposal, and the like; the preventive measure was a vaccine of doubtful efficacy and frequent side effects; the net result was the rapid decline of vaccine use. With smallpox, however, for which the vaccine was very effective and side effects rare, there was a lag period of almost 25 years in the United States between its disappearance and the discontinuation of vaccination. It is apparent that in the streptococcal-rheumatic fever field we are still a long way from such a happy conclusion. The lessons that Sanford drew from the meeting are moderate: no drastic change in strategy. There should be greater selectivity in targeting: for instance, one could limit treatment of streptococcal sore throat to ages five and 17 years, since before five rheumatic fever is so rare, and since over 17 streptococcal infections themselves are uncommon, and both rheumatic fever and glomerulonephritis are rare. One should forget about screening asymptomatic subjects. One should eliminate follow-up cultures. One should emphasize the appropriateness of stopping oral antibiotics when culture results are negative. Don't worry about false-negative throat cultures. As for research goals, the major remaining one is a method to distinguish infections from carriage.

So the meeting ended. A group photograph was taken. Many remarked that it had been a long time since so many of the convened experts had gotten together; perhaps since the Warren Air Force Base reunion for Rammelkamp's retirement or since the second Minneapolis rheumatic fever meeting, organized by Wannamaker in 1972. More importantly, when would a similar meeting take place again, if ever? And, considering the fact that the participants were mostly in a state of advanced middle age, how many would still be living, or interested in the streptococcus?

Of all the statements at the meeting, the most important seemed to be that rheumatic fever is *still* decreasing, and that it is approaching the vanishing point. Inevitably, this will affect the allocation of public resources and the behavior of most physicians, though the risk of treating a streptococcal sore throat is not yet greater than that of not treating it. Although many areas had been reviewed, a true consensus had not been reached. But the complexity of the issues had been appreciated and the subtlety of the management decision process highlighted. Most of us went home thinking that, at least for the foreseeable future, the chagrin factor is more important than iatromathematics.

---

Note: An abridged version of these notes may appear concomitantly in *Federazione Medica*, Turin, in Italian translation.

Post-scriptum:
LEWIS WANNAMAKER, M.D.
In Memoriam

A few weeks after this meeting was held, and a few days after these notes were written, Lewis Wannamaker died, suddenly and unexpectedly, on Thursday, March 24, 1983, in St. Mathews, South Carolina, where he had been born 59 years earlier.

Lewis Wannamaker's was in many ways an exemplary life, and although we are all shocked and saddened by his death, we cannot really feel sorry for him. He was blessed by a keen intellect, a warm heart, a loving and beautiful wife, four children, and innumerable students, friends, and admirers all over the world. He was, I would venture to say, by common consent the best of us, that is the best of that motley band of physicians and scientists who had made the streptococcus and the diseases it causes their main field of study, work, vocation, or avocation, as the case may be. Early in life he became justly famous for his studies on the epidemiology and preventability of rheumatic fever, which earned him and his coworkers the Lasker award, and, more important, earned life and health for innumerable patients. Unlike many of us, he stuck to the streptococcus and the diseases it causes, and his lab in Minneapolis became a fountainhead of observations, insights, experiments, and discoveries on the microbiology, the immunology, the genetics, and the epidemiology of this fascinating organism. His students, many of whom have themselves become leaders and developed *their* students, carry on the work.

I never had the good fortune to work in the lab with Lewis Wannamaker, and this is one of my regrets; but I have know him for almost thirty years in person, and a bit longer on paper, since I read his early works before immigrating to America in the summer of 1952, and our paths crossed many times, lecturing from the same lectern, visiting each other's school, exchanging streptococcal materials from our deep freezes, and opinions, and drafts of statements put out by the various committees we chaired or served on. Throughout all this I considered him a friend, and I hope he considered me one, and this is one of my joys.

*—Angelo Taranta, M.D.*

# 22

# Denouement:
# Thoughts of an Interested Observer

*Floyd W. Denny, M.D.*

## INTRODUCTION

Markowitz opened the conference with a thoughtful and provocative summary of what has happened to the streptococcus/rheumatic fever arena since 1950. He described the temporal phases through which our understanding of the management of this organism-disease complex has passed, from one of discovery, through a time of dissemination of knowledge and finally to the time we find ourselves now, one of dissonance—the reason for this conference. The questions he raised formed the basis for and set the tone of the remainder of the conference. I have been asked by Dr. Shulman, the chairman of this conference, to "synthesize from the data presented at the conference your thoughts regarding the issues raised." The conference was organized so that four different, but overlapping topics were addressed: (1) the risk and incidence of rheumatic fever; (2) the diagnosis of pharyngitis; (3) the management of streptococcal pharyngitis; and (4) the roles of algorithms and decision analysis in the management of pharyngitis. I shall give my thoughts, and I might add my opinions, in the same sequence. The reader should keep in mind that there was no effort to get a consensus during the conference, so the ideas I express do not reflect necessarily those of the conference members.

RISK AND INCIDENCE OF RHEUMATIC FEVER

The papers by Gordis and Bisno document well that the incidence of rheumatic fever in Baltimore and Memphis has declined sharply in the last few decades, to the point that the risk of developing rheumatic fever in these areas is very small indeed. Anecdotal reports from both pediatricians and internists present confirmed these data from diverse geographical areas of the United States. Thus, there seems to be little doubt that this disease is being diagnosed infrequently in this country today.

Several nagging and/or unanswered questions and problems remain, however. The largest, and probably most important of these is: What is responsible for this decline? No data are available regarding the incidence of group A streptococcal pharyngitis, but it seemed clear from the discussion that strep infections continue to occur with a frequency that is probably not declining and certainly with a frequency that is out of line with the decline of rheumatic fever. The time over which the decrease in rheumatic fever incidence has been noted is too short for the host to have been altered sufficiently for the decline to have a genetic explanation. No data are available that demonstrate that the group A streptococcus is less rheumatogenic today than previously, but this is an attractive hypothesis held by some researchers. This then leaves some element in the environment for consideration, especially poverty, which includes such things as crowding, state of nutrition, and poor access to medical care. Indeed, data presented at the conference suggest that the environment might be important in this regard and that certain manifestations of or changes in the environment are responsible for the rheumatic fever decline, especially the adequate management of streptococcal pharyngitis.

It is my opinion that problems also remain in the diagnosis of rheumatic fever. There was some discussion that suggested that the rheumatic fever occurring now is mild and is manifested mostly by arthritis, fever, and an increase in acute phase reactants. This raised the question of whether or not the Jones Criteria need further revision; this question remains unanswered. The possibility is suggested, however, that some rheumatic fever is not being recognized now and raises the need for some up-to-date surveys of the prevalence of rheumatic heart disease in high-risk populations. In this regard, I have been puzzled in recent years by the frequent diagnosis of mitral valve prolapse in children and wonder how much of what was diagnosed in past years as rheumatic mitral valve disease

was in error, leading to falsely high estimates of the incidence of rheumatic heart disease.

Although it seems clear that rheumatic fever is disappearing rapidly from the United States, it should be stressed that this disease continues to be a problem in other
parts of the world, especially in underdeveloped countries.
Opinions were expressed that it may be declining in these
countries as well, but definitive data to document this are
lacking. The remainder of the conference was devoted to
the issues of the management of streptococcal infections in
the United States and any conclusions reached are not
necessarily applicable to other geographic areas.

## THE DIAGNOSIS OF PHARYNGITIS

I believe the primary care clinician would be well advised to
study the data summarized by the various discussants in
this section, which addressed the status of diagnostic tools
in pharyngitis. Wannamaker outlined beautifully the clinical
and epidemiological aspects of streptococcal pharyngitis.
While there are unquestioned weaknesses in using these
methods for diagnosis, they are, in my opinion, frequently
helpful and often overlooked or ignored. An interesting
sidelight of this presentation was a discussion of streptococcosis, a concept that stressed the variation in age-
related manifestations of streptococcal infections, presented
by Powers and Boisvert in 1944. While it is well recognized
that group A streptococcal infections are relatively unusual
during the first two years of life and that the infected
newborn may have few if any symptoms, the recognition of
subacute disease in the two- to three-year old, character-
ized by low grade fever and adenopathy, is extremely rare
today. Several older members of the conference suggested
also that this manifestation of streptococcosis may have been
unusual in the 1940s in areas of the United States other
than New Haven.

The presentations by Cochi et al. and Gerber outlined
the status of the throat culture as a diagnostic tool and
described a variety of techniques that are being studied to
increase the accuracy and decrease the cost of the throat
culture, and to reduce the time for the clinician to receive
results. The discussion of this subject was prompted, in
part, by reports from different laboratories that show
varying degrees of efficiency of the throat culture as a
diagnostic tool. Suggestions were made that these differences may be due, at least in part, to variations in agar
bases or strains of streptococci; the researcher involved in

such investigations would be well advised to keep this in mind.

It is clear that the throat culture is a widely used diagnostic tool. Data were presented, however, that showed that clinicians might not be using this tool well. In one study, 40% of physicians did not stop a previously prescribed antibiotic even when the culture showed no streptococci! This is a sobering statistic and suggests that primary care clinicians need to reevaluate their use of throat cultures, especially their understanding and use of negative results. There are limitations to the throat culture as a diagnostic tool. The cost is substantial, negative cultures are obtained in a small percentage of infected patients, and there is a delay in obtaining results that complicates patient management. I could detect no great enthusiasm, and certainly no consensus, from the conference members that the newly described diagnostic techniques under investigation should replace at this time the regular throat culture. After listening to all the discussion, I was impressed that the time-tested and relatively simple throat culture on a sheep blood agar plate is still the method of choice for the practicing physician.

Ayoub presented alternatives to the culture as diagnostic tools. Acute phase reactants such as white blood cell count, sedimentation rate and C-reactive protein, and the nitroblue tetrazolium test are unreliable and should not be used. Antibody tests, of which the antistreptolysin-0 is still the "gold standard," are good but do not help the clinician acutely because results cannot be obtained until several weeks later. Tests for streptococcal antigens by a variety of modern techniques are being studied in several laboratories. Some of these look promising and may eventually be helpful to the practicing physician. However, it would appear at this time that none are feasible alternatives to the throat culture as diagnostic tools.

All of this leads to the practicalities of the use of the various tools in the diagnosis of pharyngitis. My assessment of the state of the art is that the clinician should rely heavily on clinical and epidemiological data so that only selected patients get a throat culture to determine quantitatively the presence of group A streptococci. The interpretation of the throat culture remains a contentious issue and probably is the single most troublesome aspect of pharyngitis management.

I am indebted to Ed Kaplan for introducing me to a new word, phorology—a study of disease carriers—which was the topic of his presentation. It is well recognized that untreated patients "carry" streptococci for weeks or months

after being infected. What is not clear, however, is whether or not patients "carry" streptococci in their respiratory
tracts in the absence of any host reaction—acute illness,
antibody response, or the subsequent occurrence of sequelae, such as rheumatic fever and nephritis. Kaplan
believes that there is a benign carrier state, but in my
opinion his data are not compelling. This controversy
should not deter the clinician in using the throat culture.
Several qualities of the "carrier" state are documented and
need to be stressed:

1. The positivity of the throat culture decreases with time
   following initial infection, hence the necessity of doing
   quantitative throat cultures.
2. The contagiousness of the carrier is related inversely
   to the length of time the streptococcus has been
   carried.
3. Suppurative complications are more common with acute
   infections than with carriage.
4. Rheumatic fever occurs within three to five weeks
   following *onset* of a streptococcal infection. Thus,
   carriage past this point is less dangerous to the host.

Using this knowledge, the clinician should attempt to
relate the positive culture to the time that the patient
acquired the streptococcus. This can be aided by epidemiological and clinical factors and, to some extent, by the
quantitative throat culture. If it is determined that the
streptococcus was acquired within days or even several
weeks before the culture was taken, the clinician has more
reason to use an antibiotic than if the time-frame is longer.
Although in some instances this remains a tough clinical
problem, I have been impressed with the helpfulness of
these guidelines.

## MANAGEMENT OF STREPTOCOCCAL PHARYNGITIS

Dillon and Eickhoff evaluated the specific antimicrobial
treatment of streptococcal pharyngitis, including the drugs
of choice, routes and duration of administration, adverse
reactions, and certain factors that might affect the efficacy
of the antibiotic, such as compliance and penicillinase-
producing microorganisms in the pharynx. Penicillin G
remains the antibiotic of choice and injectable benzathine
penicillin is the "gold standard." Theoretically, oral penicillin should be as good, provided the patient takes the
medicine. Education of the patient (or parent in the case

of a small child) is important in this regard and has been demonstrated to increase complicance significantly. The duration of oral administration of penicillin remains a puzzling issue. Several studies have shown that ten days is more effective than shorter periods in eradicating the streptococcus. The question remains whether or not this period is required to prevent rheumatic fever. Until more data are obtained on this subject, I believe the physician should treat patients for ten days. Adverse reactions to penicillin do not seem to be a significant problem and apparently have not increased over the years.

Penicillin G should be used in all patients except those allergic to it. Erythromycin is the drug of second choice, and apparently all preparations are equally effective in treating streptococcal infections. Should a patient be allergic to both penicillin and erythromycin, one of the cephalosporins can be used.

The role of penicillinase-producing organisms in the pharynx, including *Staphylococcus aureus* and some anaerobes, remains a bit controversial. This would not appear to be a significant problem; and until further data are available, penicillin G should remain the treatment of choice in most patients.

Several publications in the past few years have reported rather high failure rates in penicillin-treated patients. The reasons for this are not clear, but I was interested in the speculation by one discussant that this may be due to better techniques for isolation of the streptococcus and not to any increased failure of penicillin to eradicate the organism.

## ROLE OF ALGORITHMS AND DECISION ANALYSIS

The papers by Feinstein, Tompkins, and Pantell left me in more of a quandary than did the rest of the conference. They discussed the role of algorithms and decision analysis, which are "new" approaches to the management of pharyngitis; the reader is well advised to study these carefully. Although I have some reservations about these approaches, I believe they deserve thoughtful consideration. Feinstein, in his inimitable way, pointed out the logic and problems of algorithms and decision analysis. The studies reported by Tompkins were all done in adult populations and are not applicable to children. The pediatrician and family physician should take heed. It seems to me that all clinicians use their own algorithms for many clinical entities (though maybe not consciously), and I believe this is good. As pointed out by Tompkins, algorithms make clinicians examine their approach to clinical management, help standardize clinical care, and are useful educational tools. Regardless of what one thinks about algorithms as such, it is clear that some patients are more at risk than others to streptococcal pharyngitis and should be managed by different ground rules. This requires that every primary care physician examine the way he/she is approaching this problem.

The issues involved in decision analysis are even more complex, it seems to me. It is hard for me to accept that the real "bottom line" in the management of patients is the monetary factor, although this is obviously important. I am concerned too that decisions have to be made with insufficient or even inaccurate data. In spite of my concerns and reservations, I do not doubt that decision analysis is a valuable tool and that we will be using it more in the future. In my opinion, the conclusions reached by Pantell regarding the specifics of the management of streptococcal infections are sound, and I recommend these to the reader.

SYNTHESIS AND SUMMARY

1.  The incidence of rheumatic fever has decreased sharply in the United States; at the same time, streptococcal pharyngitis remains a problem. The reasons for the decline are not known, but antibiotic treatment of patients with streptococcal infections may be an important factor. This dictates that we should continue to treat streptococcal pharyngitis with antibiotics until we have more information regarding this decrease. It also suggests, however, that we should examine critically the strategies for the management of streptococcal pharyngitis.

2.  The clinician should consider the available management techniques and by using them in an organized way, culture only selected patients and treat only those who have a positive streptococcus culture or those who are at high risk of having an infection.

3.  Epidemiological and clinical tools can be very helpful to the clinician and should be used in choosing patients who are at risk of having streptococcal infections and who need a throat culture.

4.  The throat culture on sheep blood agar remains the method of choice for identifying the patient with streptococci in the throat. Newer and more sophisticated diagnostic procedures are not indicated for

general use at this time.

5. It is important to distinguish the carrier from the recently infected individual, and this can be done relatively well by epidemiological and clinical observations and the quantitative throat culture.

6. Acutely ill or recently infected patients should be treated for ten days with penicillin G, unless allergic to that antibiotic. If treatment is started before culture results are known, and if the culture is negative for streptococci, antibiotic treatment should be stopped unless there is compelling reason to continue.

7. The management of streptococcal pharyngitis is in a state of flux and may very well change as new data are obtained over the next few years. The clinician should be aware of this, keep an open mind, and alter approaches to management as these data indicate changes should be made.

# Index

# About the Editor

Dr. Stanford T. Shulman is Professor of Pediatrics at Northwestern University Medical School and Chief of the Division of Infectious Diseases at the Children's Memorial Hospital in Chicago, Illinois. Dr. Shulman graduated from the University of Chicago School of Medicine in 1976 and served his pediatric residency and chief residency at the University of Chicago's Wyler Children's Hospital from 1967–1970. After a short stint as a research fellow at the Institute for Child Health and Hospital for Sick Children, Great Ormand Street, London, England, Dr. Shulman was a fellow in Pediatric Infectious Diseases and Immunology with Dr. Elia Ayoub at the University of Florida in Gainesville from 1970–1973. After serving on the faculty of the Department of Pediatrics at the University of Florida from 1973–1979, Dr. Shulman assumed his current appointments. In addition, he served as Acting Chairman of the Department of Pediatrics at Northwestern University Medical School and Pediatrician-in-Chief at the Children's Memorial Hospital from 1981–1983. Since 1980, Dr. Shulman has been Chairman of the American Heart Association's Committee on Rheumatic Fever and Bacterial Endocarditis. Dr. Shulman is the author of over 65 articles and book chapters dealing with topics related to infectious diseases in children. His research interests have been related primarily to streptococcal diseases. Dr. Shulman is married to the former Claire Zaner, and their three children are Deborah, Elizabeth, and Edward.